Quality Clini
Health (

CW00972369

Quality Clinical Supervision in the Health Care Professions:
Principled approaches to practice

Della Fish MA, MEd, PhD

Honorary Research Fellow of Exeter University, lately Principal Lecturer in Education at Brunel University School of Education; formerly West London Institute, UK

Sheila Twinn BA(Hons), PhD, RHV, RGN, RSCN

Senior Lecturer, Department of Nursing, Faculty of Medicine, The Chinese University of Hong Kong; formerly Lecturer, Department of Nursing Studies, King's College, University of London, UK

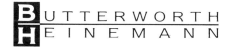

Butterworth-Heinemann
Linacre House, Jordan Hill, Oxford OX2 8DP
A division of Reed Educational and Professional Publishing Ltd

R̃ A member of the Reed Elsevier plc group

OXFORD   BOSTON   JOHANNESBURG
MELBOURNE   NEW DELHI   SINGAPORE

First published 1997

© Reed Educational and Professional Publishing Ltd 1997

British Library Cataloguing in Publication Data
A catalogue record for this book is available from the
British Library

Library of Congress Cataloguing in Publication Data
A catalogue record for this book is available from the
Library of Congress

ISBN 0 7506 2615 1

Printed and bound in Great Britain by
Biddles Ltd, Guildford and Kings Lynn

Contents

Acknowledgements

We acknowledge with gratitude the following help and support which have resulted in the preparation of this publication.

Particularly we acknowledge David Fulton, publishers, and their kind permission to base this book on Della Fish's *Quality Mentoring for Student Teachers: a principled approach to practice*, which was published in 1995.

In addition we thank all our colleagues (staff and students) in the range of health care professions with which we are associated, and from whom we have learnt so much about clinical supervision. For their particular help we thank: Carol Daglish, Sarah Forester, Crissie Gallagher, Hazel Harrison and Anne Palmer.

This book would not have reached the publisher without the dedication of Jean Douglas and Evelyn Usher who with endless patience and good humour meticulously corrected drafts and proofread, nor without Susan Devlin, commissioning editor for Butterworth-Heinemann, who brought a human touch to her role in liaising with us.

Any opinions expressed are entirely ours and are in no way associated with any institution or official body for which either of us works.

Della Fish and Sheila Twinn

Glossary

BAAB	British Acupuncture Accreditation Board
BAcC	British Acupuncture Council
BMA	British Medical Association
CCAM	Council for Complementary and Alternative Medicine
CNAA	Council for National Academic Awards
CNO	Chief Nursing Officer
COT	College of Occupational Therapists
CPSM	Council for Professions Supplementary to Medicine
CSP	Chartered Society of Physiotherapists
DES	Department of Education and Science
DHA	District Health Authority
DMU	Directly Managed Unit
DoH	Department of Health
ENB	English National Board for Nursing, Midwifery and Health Visiting
FHSA	Family Health Service Authority
GNVQ	General National Vocational Qualification
HE	Higher Education
HMI	Her Majesty's Inspector
HMSO	Her Majesty's Stationery Office
HVA	Health Visitors Association
IPR	Individual Performance Review
ITE	Initial Teacher Education
LSA	Local Supervising Authority
MPE	Multiprofessional Education
NCVQ	National Council for Vocational Qualifications
NDU	Nursing Development Unit
NFER	National Foundation for Educational Research
NHS	National Health Service
NHSE	National Health Service Executive
NHSME	National Health Service Management Executive
NVQ	National Vocational Qualification

OT   Occupational Therapy/Therapist
PA (model) Professional Artistry (model)
PREP   Post Registration Education and Practice
PT   Physiotherapy/Physiotherapist
RHA   Regional Health Authority
TR (model) Technical–Rational (model)
UK   United Kingdom
UKCC   United Kingdom Central Council for Nursing, Midwifery
            and Health Visiting

Introduction

The context and the readership

The increasing importance of clinical supervision for student practitioners – and now for qualified practitioners – has been highlighted by the complexities that currently pervade health care provision within the National Health Service (NHS) and through the work towards government recognition by those professions presently unregulated, like acupuncture and herbal medicine which are currently seen as alternative to, or complementary to, western medicine.

However, the reasons for the increased significance of clinical supervision appear on the surface to vary. For example, in professions aspiring to government recognition, the quality of supervision depends upon its *educational* role in enabling the student to learn *through* as well as *from* practice (see below, p. 80). Whereas, in nursing, supervision is now no longer only for those aspiring to join a profession, but is seen as equally appropriate for qualified practitioners, which might (erroneously, we believe in company with many) suggest rather a managerial than an educational role for the supervisor.

Yet, in spite of its increasing significance and the consequent growth in demand for quality supervisors, as far as we are aware there are no books on clinical supervision which are focused explicitly on the needs of health care professionals.

This is not to overlook the literature from nursing including the King's Fund publication on nursing, the United Kingdom Central Council for nursing, midwifery and health visiting's (UKCC's) position statement on clinical supervision (UKCC, 1996a) and the work of Butterworth and Faugier on clinical supervision (Butterworth and Faugier, 1992; Faugier and Butterworth, 1993), or Chris Johns' work on professional supervision (Johns, 1993) and reflective practice (Johns, 1994, 1995) and White and Ewan (1991). Neither is it to ignore Stengelhofen's *Teaching Students in Clinical Settings* (1993) or the writing from social work, and counselling and psychotherapy (e.g. Hawkins and Shohet's *Supervision in the Helping Professions,* 1989) as well as the work of Alsop and Ryan aimed at occupational therapy students (Alsop and Ryan, 1996). We are also, as will be clear from our text, well aware of and draw heavily upon the literature from teaching (see bibliography at the back of this book).

We would claim, however, that this book is considerably unlike most of these. Not only is it directed at all readers in health care professions, but it is also different in four other ways which we believe to be significant.

It differs first in that it is addressed to **members of professions across** *both* **western** *and* **oriental approaches to health care**, and specifically it addresses those professionals who work with students or colleagues to enable them to learn or refine the practice of their profession.

In using the term 'health care professions', then, we intend to include all those occupations whose dedication to the service of (the good of, or the health or nurture of) their clients and society at large is pre-eminent. We take the word professional to be a proper accolade where the work is 'esoteric, complex, discretionary', and can only be learnt during 'a demanding period of training'; where there is commitment to practising an agreed and regulated body of knowledge and skill of special value; and where a fiduciary relationship (a trust by the client of the professional which depends upon public confidence) is maintained with clients (Freidson, 1994, p. 200). Such professions are either already recognized by Act of Parliament, or will be working towards gaining such recognition or aiming at self-regulation.

In using the term 'clinical supervision' we mean the work carried out in the arena of professional practice by a qualified practitioner working with a student who is learning to become a professional or (in some professions) with a professional who is seeking to develop and refine his or her practice. We are aware that some professions define supervision itself very broadly (see for example College of Occupational Therapists (COT, 1990)), but our work focuses on the **educational** and **professional development** aspects of clinical supervision.

There are, as we are also aware, many different terms for what we shall call clinical supervision, and, as we said in 1990 (Fish, Twinn and Purr, 1990, p. 3), their very existence indicates that there is amazingly little cross-profession deliberation about these matters. We are also aware of the aversion in nursing for the term 'supervisor' when used for work with qualified practitioners, but we use it here because it is still the most common term for this work and because our definition of supervisor – whomever the supervisor works with – is not that of 'overseeing manager' but of 'educational collaborator'.

We are also aware that in different professions the 'fieldwork' or practical element of the professional preparation course is in a different relationship with the theoretical work, and that this even involves a different physical relationship of practice and theory, which itself is a sign of deeper issues which are significant for the supervisor. For example, while those learning to become occupational therapists and physiotherapists must be placed in a range of hospital and community settings often at quite a distance from their theoretical course, and nurses are now educated in colleges of nursing associated with universities to which are usually related a group of hospitals, in acupuncture the clinic at which patients are treated is usually attached to the college itself. These differing settings make for differing demands upon the supervisor and on preparation offered to the supervisor.

Despite these differences, however, we believe that in writing about clinical supervision we are raising issues, considering principles and discussing practices which are relevant to all professional practitioners whose role involves the supervision of the practice of either students learning to become professionals or fellow professionals seeking to develop and improve their practice. Because we believe that the educational principles are the same no matter what the care or therapy for which the professional is being educated, we have the temerity to offer our material to, for example, those in the **nursing profession**, and also to **chiropodists, dieticians, occupational therapists, orthoptists, physiotherapists, and radiographers**, as well as to those in the emerging professions of, for example, **acupuncture, homeopathy, osteopathy,** and **phytotherapy (herbal medicine)**. What holds all such professions together despite differences of direction about cure, palliative care, therapy or nurture, is that they are professionals dedicated to the physical and mental good of their clients and needing to be educated as professional practitioners. Thus we believe that there is much to be gained by those in health care professions in recognizing that they share the same educational intentions, realizing that they are working on the same problems and talking together and learning from each other about shared issues.

Secondly, what we offer here is a different view of professionalism from that found in much current literature. We regard the practice of the professional, and therefore of the clinical supervisor, as a matter not of learning prescribed skills and applying them efficiently to practice, but of developing understanding and providing support in refining professional judgement. In other words, whatever the individual profession involved, a clinical supervisor is an educator, and bears responsibility (for which he or she is rarely specially prepared) for a major aspect of professional development. Thus this book is different in that it sees clinical supervision as rooted firmly in education rather than in training and regards the clinical supervisor as an agent of professional development rather than as a control mechanism.

Thirdly, we offer a different interpretation of the notion of quality from that found in many current publications. We see quality as arising from sound education and the endless search for self-improvement which is the hallmark of a professional. We recognize that this differs considerably from the currently prevalent view that quality arises either from the imposition of targets from outside a profession or (as in nursing) from the professionals themselves who have become standard setters for their own profession. It is also different from self-improvement in that these standards, once met, are endlessly raised for reasons which are often more to do with finance than education or service. We also seek to draw attention to, and even to challenge, the fact that this idea has become so all-pervasive that it is regarded, despite its obvious moral shortcomings, as the only view that professionals can have.

Fourthly, unlike much of the current professional literature in professions supplementary to western medicine, and also in some literature in the oriental traditions, where it is assumed that the professional will simply accept the situation which currently obtains, and imbue supervisees with the same accepting attitude, we seek to heighten the critical awareness and critical consciousness of professionals in respect of their professional work, their professionalism and the profession to which they belong. Indeed, we believe that a further mark of a professional is an ability to think independently and exercise professional judgement not only about the work with clients but also about the professional and social context, the values, the assumptions made about professional matters and matters of wider significance which affect professionals generally. Of course, this view brings with it a corresponding idea about how the clinical supervisor ought to work with the professional colleague for whom he or she has an educational responsibility.

The focus of this book, then, is different from previous books on clinical supervision in the following three respects:

1 It views the enterprise of learning to be a professional as concerned with learning to be a member of a profession rather than as merely learning to be an individually operating, proficient practitioner.
2 It therefore sees the intentions of clinical supervision as educating students to become members of a profession rather than as training them to be deliverers of a government or private sector service or an alternative to these.
3 It seeks to prepare quality clinical supervisors by offering them education rather than training.

The material offered here, therefore, seeks to work towards quality clinical supervision, through *education*, rather than training. We therefore offer a basis for both discussing some central issues and establishing some principles and also for trying out and considering professional and clinical supervision practices. What we do *not* offer is a blue-print for good supervision. To paraphrase what Alexander says of good practice, one could say that quality health care practice and quality clinical supervision (indeed, quality professional development generally) are not achieved through rhetoric and decree or bureaucratic will and government control, but 'dialectically and empirically' *in practice* (Alexander, 1990, p. 72). Neither are they about learning pre-ordained skills and applying them.

Thus, in order to provide a basis for its twin concerns about principles and practices, this book focuses on, or will help readers to focus on:

- the traditions and the present knowledge-base of the supervisor's profession (using as exemplars teacher education and nursing simply because here is where there is most literature on supervision)
- the complex character of health care practice and the social traditions of each profession
- the nature of the wider professional perspectives characteristic of a member of a profession
- techniques of investigation and reflection which enable professionals to refine health care practice and professional activity.

In doing so it offers:

- experience of what is involved in learning through practice, ways of enabling students to learn through practice, and analysis of such experience
- consideration of the strengths and weaknesses of various activities associated with observation, debriefing, assessment
- experience in articulating and considering ethically the personal theory that underlies professional action, and of enabling students to do so
- experience in uncovering, scrutinizing and thinking ethically about the principles and grounds of professional action, and of providing support for students doing so.

And in all this, it invites response from the reader throughout by offering during each chapter a series of reflection points to consider and tasks to work on, alone or with a colleague.

This work is directed at the individual supervisor but it might also be used as a basis for professional development sessions on more formal and collegiate occasions. It is interactive. In raising issues and enabling readers to consider educational principles, it draws upon the extensive knowledge-base of initial teacher education, its research and traditions, especially as developed in recent decades, and upon the work of nursing, and it invites members of other professions to search out and supply the detail available from their own context.

There is much that has been written for teachers on mentoring student teachers (mentors being equivalent to clinical supervisors) because there has been a major move in the last 5 years to place teacher 'training' in the hands of school teachers and to move it substantially out of higher education. But, although the opposite move has been and is being made in many of the health care professions – namely to bring the preparation for entry to them into higher education – and although professional bodies have produced documents containing requirements in respect of practical work in these preparation courses, there is relatively little in print which seeks to support clinical supervision by educating the supervisor, and most of what there is, is not in book form available to 'fieldworkers' who lack ready access to academic journals.

The other literature and practices which we highlight are those from nursing where the role of clinical supervisor has been considerably extended to include a professional development role where the supervisor works with a qualified practitioner. Two major influences have contributed to these recent developments in nursing. The first relates to government policy documents in respect of that profession and the second to the rather more general demand for excellence in practice which comes from government initiatives and also from within the profession, where, for example, the UKCC has developed principles for clinical supervision in nursing and health visiting (UKCC 1996a). Policy documents such as the National Health Service Management Executive's (NHSME) publication, *A Vision for the Future* (NHSME, 1993b) identified 12 key targets for the contribution of nursing, midwifery and health visiting to health care. Two of these targets focus specifically on clinical supervision. The Department of Health (DoH) in England has also targeted more specific areas of practice such as child protection, where clinical supervision is seen as essential for high quality care and developed a resource pack for clinical supervision (NHSE, 1995).

The intentions

This book, then, is offered in the belief that clarification of one's uncertainties about professional practice and a willingness to investigate, reflect upon and refine one's theories and practices is a better base from which to work with students and colleagues than the unfounded and quickly punctured certainty that springs from ignorance of the complexities. It is addressed therefore to those who seek rather than those who consider that they know. In offering an educational foundation for clinical supervision it challenges the skills-based training approach of much current literature.

Its intentions are to enable readers to:

• recognize the problematic nature of professional practice
• have an open mind about their own practice and theories
• become experienced in reflecting on their own practice
• know how to continue to investigate and refine practice and theory
• be able to articulate their personal philosophical approach to professional practice
• be ready to enable students to articulate their own personal approach to professional practice and to find their own ways of operating successfully in practice
• have a clear idea of how they want to operate as clinical supervisors
• know how their supervision relates to work done with students in higher education.

In short, this book is directed at setting the feet of clinical supervisors on a path towards a principled approach to practice, built upon the twin foundations of seeking better understanding of issues and continual refinement of practice, and having, as a central characteristic, a view of quality which rests upon professional insight (evidenced by wise practice and sound professional judgements), rather than on the measurement of required visible behaviour.

The rationale

The rationale for the book springs from comparing two broad views about teaching and learning to teach.

One view (**the technical–rational view**) is that practice is a simple set of competencies which can be learnt by the practitioner and the supervisor. Here the supervisor needs to learn skills and strategies of counselling, observing and assessing of the kind most frequently found in courses for the education and training of practitioners in health care. It is assumed that, having learnt these skills and strategies, the supervisor will merely have to apply them in practice in order to supervise the practitioner. The skills and strategies enshrined in the technical–rational views are relatively simple to learn (though the professional judgement about when and how to operate them is more difficult than its proponents admit). This approach certainly offers one starting point for supervision in times of limited resources, but some people have reservations about its educational qualities and its longer term advantages.

The other view (**the reflective practitioner view**) is that practice is a complex, dynamic, social activity underpinned by sets of values and beliefs, traditions and theoretical perspectives, and with a moral dimension. In this case supervising the practitioner involves the supervisor in:

- acknowledging and trying to understand this complexity
- seeking to articulate and keep under review a clear principled base to personal practice (even if that means recognizing that the context of practice may make this a complex process)
- knowing how research can enlighten professional practice
- knowing how to investigate practice, how to unearth the theory from it and how to reflect upon it, theorize about it and challenge it with formal theory
- understanding how individual practice relates to the moral and the traditional aspects of professional practice and recognizing the implications of this for supervision
- being able to draw out the ideas, beliefs, assumptions and values that lie at the base of the practitioner's practice
- being able to help the practitioner to find new approaches to practice and their underpinning rationales
- being able to help the practitioner find his or her own preferred approach to professional practice
- being able to engage in discussions with the practitioner about the purposes of health care, in order to enable the practitioner to explore how his or her own practice relates to the values and beliefs determining the different approaches to care.

The reflective practitioner view of supervising practitioners is more demanding than the technical–rational approach. It requires a greater degree of intellectual and professional time and energy and a willingness to work at articulating the professional knowledge which practitioners traditionally draw upon in practice but often find hard to put into words. That is, it requires more of supervisors than merely directing and evaluating or assessing practice. In addition, it takes more effort and greater resources to prepare such supervisors. However, it offers practitioner and supervisor a learning adventure in which each can contribute to the growth of the other in an infinite variety of ways and which will enable practitioners to take responsibility for their own continued development.

The aim of this book is therefore to explore these two different approaches to supervision and to enable supervisors to develop a reflective practice approach not only to supervision but also to practice. To achieve this aim the following intentions have been identified:

- to develop an understanding of the process of reflecting on practice
- to develop awareness of the educational responsibilities of clinical supervisors
- to enable supervisors to articulate their personal philosophical approach to their own practice and to clinical supervision
- to enable supervisors to recognize the problematic nature of practice in health care
- to enable supervisors to have an open mind about their own practices and theories
- to enable supervisors to continue to investigate and refine theories and processes of supervision and practice.

The structure

The book is offered in three parts. **The *first* part** deals with a range of issues that all supervisors need to appreciate if their work is to be of high quality. Each chapter considers a key issue. These are:

- contextual issues for supervision (an understanding of the scope of professional practice and what factors influence its current character)
- key views of professionalism that influence current thinking about practice generally and affect individual activities in the practice setting
- the processes and responsibilities of supervision.

For each issue a range of differing approaches and views is considered, some practical investigations are offered for supervisors to carry out alone or with a colleague, the influence of the practice setting is considered and some further reading is recommended.

The *second* part focuses specifically on the practice of supervision. It considers how supervisors might enable practitioners to develop proficiency in practice, and promote their understanding of the deeper issues that influence their work. It also offers ideas on how supervisors might draw practitioners to investigate their practice, and develop it and refine it. This section begins with a chapter on notions of good practice – which are central to views on supervision. Later chapters focus on the evaluation of practice, including debriefing the practitioner. For each aspect a range of differing approaches and views is considered, some practical investigations are offered for supervisors to carry out alone or with a colleague, the influence of the practice setting is considered and some further reading is recommended as follow up.

The *third* **part** considers the important wider role of the supervisor which is often neglected or treated very superficially. This section looks at how the supervisor can help the practitioner develop his or her level of professionalism rather than simply become a proficient performer in practice. This involves supporting the practitioner in his or her investigations of practice-based issues as well as exploring some of the organizational issues which have implications for practice and professional matters.

Postscript

This book is about quality supervision as opposed to supervisor training. To ignore the first and last parts of this book would be to ignore the very issues that distinguish the quality supervisor from the trained supervisor. Readers are therefore advised not simply to skip to the practical chapters but to read the text in chronological order.

Della Fish and Sheila Twinn

Part One

*Quality clinical supervision:
understanding the enterprise*

1

The context for supervision: establishing a sound base for practice

Introduction

The notion of quality in health care provision has become linked in most professions now with an increased significance in the role of the clinical supervisor. It is the educational aspects of such a role with which we are concerned in this publication. We are aware of the European Community's 1995 White Paper on Education and Training, with its focus on building a learning society by means of European-wide systems for accrediting technical and vocational skills and the notion that ultimately everyone will carry a 'personal skills card'. However, we reject the notion that profession is the same as occupation and believe that professional preparation in the context of higher education is outside the scope of this 'base level' approach (which seems to be the inevitable result of trying to regulate learning by means of a huge bureaucratic system).

In considering professional education, then, in the context of clinical supervision for the health care professions, we seek specifically to address the following professionals: those in nursing; those in the six relevant professions which have operated within the framework of the Council for Professions Supplementary to Medicine (CPSM) – chiropody, dietetics, occupational therapy (OT), orthoptics, physiotherapy (PT) and radiotherapy – and those in the emerging professions of complementery medicine, particularly those which are members of the Council for Complementary and Alternative Medicine (CCAM) – acupuncture, homeopathy, medical herbalism, and osteopathy. In grouping the professions in this way, we recognize that the CPSM, being a *statutory* body which acts as an enabling framework and a focus for the Boards of the seven professions it serves (CPSM, 1995, p. 4), is inevitably different in nature from the CCAM which is an equally official body but which simply provides a forum for communication and cooperation between professional bodies whose professions are not yet State regulated (CCAM, 1993, p. 1). In respect of these latter professions, we note that there is an 'unprecedented expansion of complementary and alternative medicine in health care today' (Rankin-Box, 1995, p. 27), that many of them are beginning to be utilized in mainstream nursing practice, and that there is now evidence of collaboration between general and complementary practitioners (Reason, 1995). Many of these professions are in the process of seeking State regulation and are working to core syllabuses in which clinical supervision is important (e.g. British Medical Association (BMA), 1993; Fisher, 1995; Shifrin, 1995). We also note with interest the moves abroad on Multiprofessional Education (MPE) in undergraduate curricula (Davidson and Lucas, 1995), and believe that the interest in common educational goals that are professionally relevant (Davidson and Lucas, 1995, p. 164) is bound to include a focus upon clinical supervision.

In professions like OT and PT on the one hand or acupuncture and herbal medicine on the other, the role of the clinical supervisor (often called the fieldwork educator) in the preregistration course has become pivotal to securing quality preregistration preparation. Indeed, many professions, recognizing this, now offer a range of supervisor training courses, and some, like OT and community health care nursing, have been offering such courses for many years. Our contention, however, is that these usually deal with the skills required, some deal with educational understanding but few, if any, find time to consider principles in any depth.

Nursing education and practice offer an example where the growing demand for high quality care and the professional requirements for education and practice *following* registration have pushed the concept of clinical supervision to the top of the agenda. Thus, within nursing, the term clinical supervision raises some interesting questions and issues for practitioners, since it is used to refer both to the professional gatekeeping role played by supervisors during preregistration and post-registration programmes, as well as to the supervision of the professional development of qualified practitioners. (We shall use the term 'professional development' to denote the education of qualified practitioners, although we acknowledge that students too are engaged in the development of their professionalism from the start of their course.) For nursing, then, the process involved in these two different settings for clinical supervision raises questions about whether the process should be different for these two levels of practice or whether the skills and expertise required by the supervisor ought to be similar in both settings.

We believe, however, that until all professions enable supervisors to consider the principles on which they work (i.e. provide education for them), rather than simply working on their skills (i.e. training them), those supervisors in turn will not be able to educate their students or colleagues and the *professional* nature of practice will be diminished. Education frees a professional to operate appropriately in context, where training only expects the application of what has been pre-learnt. We shall be looking in detail at these matters in Chapters 2 and 3 below.

The world of nursing and health care generally is also becoming more complex, with increasing technology and complex health needs requiring increasing expertise of the practitioner. For example, the changing demands of professional education are introducing new concepts into practice with which supervisors must familiarize themselves and for which they must develop appropriate levels of expertise. The integration of higher education with nurse education has contributed to the demands for a research-based approach to practice which has contributed to the demands made of clinical supervisors. In addition the introduction of quality assurance and standard setting in practice has introduced new philosophies of care within the NHS, which may not fit easily with some philosophies of clinical supervision nor indeed the philosophy of the individual supervisor.

Such situations have, in all health care professions, created an increasingly complex structure in which the clinical supervisor has to practice. The aim of the subsequent chapters in this book is to explore some of these issues and processes. However, prior to the discussion of processes involved in clinical supervision it is important that practitioners with a responsibility for clinical supervision have an understanding of the context in which they practice. This chapter therefore aims to highlight some of the factors contributing to this contextual setting by focusing on four particular perspectives. The first of these is focused on the *intention* of clinical supervision, the second on the *historical development* of clinical supervision, the third on the *requirements* of government and professional statutory bodies and the last considers the *personal agenda* of the individual supervisor. In developing these perspectives the chapter offers an overview of some of the problematic issues in clinical supervision in nursing, providing practitioners with the opportunity to debate these issues and the implications for practice. Indeed some of the key questions it tries to address are as follows:

- What are (and what should be) the main intentions of clinical supervision?
- How has clinical supervision come to where it is now? (What can we learn from history?)
- What roles are envisaged for the supervisor and the clinical setting?
- What values are enshrined in the key government documents?
- What are the key responsibilities of being a supervisor?

- What are the government and professional statutory bodies' requirements of supervisors, students and practitioners?

Clinical supervision in a professional context

Aims and intentions of clinical supervision

In considering the aims and intentions of clinical supervision it is necessary to address what we wish to call the two different **modes** of clinical supervision. These are: **mode one, the on-course mode**, where the supervisor operates within the context of a professionally focused course, and **mode two, the professional development mode**, where the supervisor works with a qualified practitioner in the context of their daily work. They are of significance even though for some professions so far the on-course mode is the only one currently operating. In nursing at present there is a formal move to involve individual supervisors in both rather than simply one of these modes, and with the different levels of student preparation and education which occur within these. Other professions too are already moving or have moved in the direction of adopting the professional development mode, and it is therefore important that supervisors consider critically the educational aims of these two approaches to supervision as they determine consciously the philosophical basis on which they wish to work.

The first mode of clinical supervision (the on-course mode) has been well established within most professions for many years and in nursing involves the clinical supervision of students at both pre- and post-registration levels because in nursing there exists a number of levels beyond the initial qualification. As discussed later in this chapter, although the strategies and responsibilities of clinical supervision in this mode have changed and developed over the years, the aim of clinical supervision has remained constant and can be defined as that of facilitating student learning in the practice setting and assessing competence in practice. The responsibility for assessing competence in practice highlights the important gatekeeping role of supervisors in this approach to supervision. For those supervisors working with post-registration students the gatekeeping role may be modified, in that it cannot prevent the professional registration of the students, but may nevertheless prevent student practitioners from adopting their new practice role, where for example it involves preparing for the role of specialist practitioners (English National Board [ENB], 1995).

The second and much newer of these approaches involves the clinical supervision of qualified practitioners. In occupational therapy, for example, supervision itself is widely defined, but its educational focus seems to be a lesser priority than its management concerns (see below, p. 34). In acupuncture, (clinical) supervision of newly trained acupuncturists has long since been discussed and has recently been called for (McPherson, 1993, 1995). Such supervision has only recently been introduced in nursing (apart from psychiatric nursing) and its emergence and development are discussed in more detail below (p. 24). Here, despite some continuing debate about the major purpose of such supervision, resulting from the early stage of its development, the literature identifies some clearly defined aims for it. Swain (1995) suggests that an important aim of supervision is to allow practitioners to reflect on their practice in order to develop their professional expertise. Kohner (1994), in a discussion of the contribution of supervision to professional practice, argues that it provides practitioners with the opportunity to learn from experience. Some of the confusion experienced by practitioners in understanding the aim of supervision is identified in the position paper prepared by Faugier and Butterworth (1993), which gives a very comprehensive review of the concept of clinical supervision. This paper highlights the tendency to equate the term supervision with a management responsibility. The paper cites the definition provided by Butterworth (1992) which describes supervision 'as an exchange between practising professionals to enable the development of professional skills'. Within these definitions, although the different authors highlight the development of the professional practice of practitioners as a major aim of supervision, the emphasis on skills rather than the expertise of the supervisor is, in our view, a limited interpretation of supervision. We would argue that educators need to be free to make their own judgements and to exercise skills appropriate to each new context and that this is best achieved if the supervisor has first understood the principles upon which he or she intends to act.

It can be argued that the aims of these two modes of clinical supervision place a different *emphasis* on the responsibility of the supervisor. In both, however, the *role* of supervisor is seen as having major implications for the development of students' and practitioners' perception and interpretation of professional practice. It is therefore important for supervisors to establish a principled basis upon which to consider the implications of their philosophy and interpretation of practice.

Aims and professional practice

The following questions about the aims and nature of professional practice illustrate something of the complexity of these issues. As demonstrated in the discussion in later chapters, these questions are not idle philosophizing. The ways in which professional bodies, educators, politicians and managers seek to answer them gives rise to the practical arrangements currently used in clinical supervision. The ways supervisors answer them will both determine the broad approach to supervision and equip supervisors with well-thought-through responses to legitimate questions that are likely to arise from supervisees. Further, understanding this helps to explain past practice, to think analytically about present initiatives and may even help in clarifying the range of hopes for the future.

Task 1.1 Preparation for reflection
(alone or with a colleague)

1 Offer your own answers to the questions in the main text below.
2 Explore your replies to see what values and priorities lie underneath them.
3 Consider your own professional philosophies.
4 If possible share your findings with a colleague.

Preliminary comment
We do not always know what it is we personally value until we come up against such questions, and then we may be disconcerted that there are conflicts between what we say and what we do, or even between our preferred answer to one question and another.
   But at least to recognize these is:

• to have unearthed matters that will repay further exploration
• to know more about how we wish to respond to questions about practice aims
• to have the power to challenge, refine, develop or change our ideas
• to begin to develop or to refine continuously our own overall practice philosophy
• to be able to discuss these ideas in an informed way with students and practitioners.

The following points are also worthy of note:

(a) Arguably, one of the tasks of clinical supervisors is to enable students and practitioners to explore their values and their own philosophy of professional practice and professionalism.
(b) Equally it is important that those working with students or practitioners do not consider that they know and have 'cracked' these things. Certainty about such matters arises only from ignorance about their complexity, and is a sure way of stopping student learning or further professional development dead in its tracks.
(c) You may wish to return to and revise your responses to the questions in the light of later parts of the book.

Some questions about professional practice

Although these questions relate specifically to the supervision of students, they are also relevant to the supervision of qualified practitioners.

1 What do practitioners need to know? Should clinical supervision aim to equip students with only that which is necessary to deliver safe care in a particular practice setting or should it also educate them about their wider role as a health care practitioner in a profession?

2 What ought to be involved in learning to be an efficient practitioner? How might this be learnt?

3 What is the relationship between what students and practitioners know and how they practice?

4 What is, or might be, involved in the wider role of the practitioner, what is involved in coming to be a full member of a profession, and how can students acquire professional knowledge?

5 How important is it to maintain the professional nature of practice and to be a member of a *profession* today? (Has the importance of professionalism been eroded by changes in views about authority and accountability? Has the meaning of 'professional' changed?)

6 Is it important that nursing should be an all-graduate profession? How important is it that practitioners should undergo a rigorous course of preregistration education which leads to validated higher education qualification?

7 What should be attempted in the short term in student preparation and education and what should be left to the longer-term continuing education and supervision?

8 How important is it that practitioners should play a significant part in defining entry standards, assessing students and evaluating courses?

9 Who should prescribe the curriculum and content for courses in professional practice?

10 What exactly is/should be higher education's contribution to professional practice? What place does a university have in the vocational and professional preparation of, for example, acupuncturists, dieticians, nurses, OTs, PTs, radiographers?

As we have already seen, there are no simple, universal answers to these questions. Yet answers to them shape clinical supervision at both student and qualified practitioner level. Further questions now arise, therefore, about how this has come to happen and about what is now required of supervision. Again, the following offers a framework which those anxious to provide quality supervision will need to be aware of in order to make sense of their own place in both history and the present.

Clinical supervision in its historical context

Professions ignore the influence of historical trends and traditions at the peril of losing their very professionalism, since all professions rest upon traditions and history, since history is one of our best ways of making sense of the present, and since it needs to be understood and considered critically if we are to make progress in the future.

It is therefore important to consider the context in which clinical supervision has developed in each profession, and to explore the development of such clinical supervision. For most professions this will mean considering our first mode of supervision (the on-course mode). In nursing, however, both modes have developed and it is interesting to observe that in each there has been a particularly significant factor influencing the development of the process of supervision. Nursing

---

**Task 1.2 Reflection on supervision for all health care
professionals except nurses**
(alone or with a colleague)

Use the following questions (and perhaps the nursing examples provided in the following few pages) to help you consider the context for clinical supervision in your own profession. Note, however, that for most professions only the on-course mode of supervision will have been operating.

1 What were the major *events* in the history of the evolution of your profession that relate to the way clinical supervision has developed? (Think analytically and critically about the history of this.)
2 What changes have been made in the last 20 years to:
   • the ways in which clinical supervision is perceived by the profession, and by students
   • how supervision relates to the rest of the course
   • the processes deemed to be central to it
   • the kind of provision made for educating or training supervisors
   • the relationship between supervision and professional development?
   How do you view these changes?
3 Is there any sign in your profession of the possible introduction of professional development supervision, and what are your views about this?

examples are used in the following pages because other professions have less full documentation to draw upon and because nursing has developed further in respect of clinical supervision. Members of other professions should now use Task 1.2 to help them consider ways of looking at the history of supervision in their own profession.

The evolution of clinical supervision in nursing

In student supervision the implementation of Project 2000, heralded as a radical new approach to nurse education, significantly changed the status of students in the practice setting, as well as the status of their educational preparation. Within the domain of qualified practitioners the publication of *A Vision for the Future* (NHSME, 1993b) raised clinical supervision to the top of the agenda in many different professional settings. These two significant events will therefore be placed in their historical setting as a means of examining the evolution of clinical supervision for nursing.

Mode 1: student supervision prior to the implementation of Project 2000

Obviously in a book such as this, it is neither appropriate nor possible to give a detailed history of clinical supervision in nurse education. It is however possible to identify some of the major factors which have influenced the process. Indeed prior to the implementation of Project 2000 clinical supervision generally was based on the traditional apprenticeship model in which an assumption was made that if students were placed in the clinical setting, they would learn the skills of nursing from working alongside other nurses. This model, which Jarvis (1983) describes as 'Sitting by Nellie', disregards the essential role of skilled supervisors in facilitating learning in the clinical setting and assumes that students will develop expertise in professional practice through natural absorption of skills and knowledge. Kenworthy and Nicklin (1989) describe student nurses at this time as spending up to 80 per cent of their preregistration courses in this learning environment. In addition, this approach to supervision also raised questions about who was the most appropriate practitioner from whom the student should 'absorb' their skills and knowledge of practice. In attempting to answer this question, responsibility for clinical supervision has moved full circle from trained ward staff in the 1940s, to practitioners employed as clinical teachers in the 1960s, to providing special training programmes in clinical teaching for qualified practitioners in the 1980s.

Whoever the practitioner responsible for clinical supervision was, however, the problem of the integration of theory and practice in the clinical setting remained. It was in response to concerns about the existing system of nurse education, as well as to the problems of service delivery (created by the system of nurse education and projected demographic changes), that prompted the radical review of nurse education in the form of Project 2000 (UKCC, 1986).

Mode 1: clinical supervision post Project 2000

The implementation of Project 2000 in 1990 changed nursing education in three major ways. First, the award of an educational higher diploma, as well as a professional qualification, has made an explicit link between higher education and nursing education. Secondly, the requirement by the professional statutory body for 50 per cent of the curriculum to be allocated to theory and 50 per cent to practice, provides an equal emphasis on these components of nurse preparation. Finally, the allocation of supernumerary status for students for the majority of the course allows them true student status and removes their contribution to the workforce. This last change has particular implications for clinical supervision since it allows students much greater opportunity for professional development during their learning experience. However, the responsibility for clinical supervision remains with practitioners in the clinical setting, and this still raises issues about the process of supervision.

One issue, in particular, is the demand created for practitioners in managing their dual responsibility of managing patient and client care and carrying out clinical supervision (Twinn and Davis, 1996). Further, in a study of the relationship between teaching, support, support and role modelling in the clinical areas, White *et al.* (1994) identified the need for clarification of the different roles of clinical staff and lecturing staff when supervising students in the practice area. The findings of the study also raise questions about what levels of clinical practice should be demonstrated by practitioners within the context of clinical supervision, when students are studying for a higher diploma. In addition, the findings of the study also demonstrated the complexities of facilitating learning in the clinical area and this highlights the expertise required by supervisors of clinical practice, which supports understandings gained during previous research (Fish, Twinn and Purr, 1991; Twinn, 1992). Project 2000 may have introduced a new approach to nurse education then, but major issues remain unresolved and require careful consideration by supervisors.

In addition to supervising students within Project 2000, many supervisors will also be involved in the supervision of qualified staff as a result of *A Vision for the Future*. Here many of the issues are similar to those described above, but there are significant additional matters to address which are created by the development of a new domain of clinical supervision. And in addressing these, the nursing profession has little cross-professional assistance to call upon.

Mode 2: clinical supervision of qualified staff prior to 1993

Prior to the publication of the new strategy for nursing, midwifery and health visiting in 1993 entitled *A Vision for the Future* (NHSME, 1993b), clinical supervision of qualified staff working in post was generally limited to two disciplines within nursing: psychiatric nursing and midwifery. In psychiatric nursing, with its focus on the 'therapeutic case of self' and the fundamental role of interpersonal skills to practice (Barker, 1992), the importance of supervision of qualified staff has been recognized for many years. Barker (1992) goes on to argue that such supervision in psychiatric nursing has two major aims, first to protect patients receiving care from nurses and secondly to protect nurses from themselves. Indeed Simms, cited in Swain (1995), demonstrates a history of commitment to supervision in this discipline of nursing since the 1940s. Although the introduction of the new syllabus for mental health nursing in 1982 provided the opportunity for supervision to become a reality for practitioners, rather than merely an idea, some authors argue that examples of supervision in practice remain few and far between, with nurses frequently only having access to informal peer support groups (Carson cited in Swain, 1995).

In midwifery a rather different approach to supervision is present with a requirement, laid down in statute in 1902, for practising midwives to receive regular supervision. This supervision, although changing through the years, remained predominantly grounded in a competency-based model of supervision.

The most recent legislation shaping this supervision is that of the Nurses, Midwives and Health Visitors Act of 1979 and 1992. Now the national boards for the education of nurses, midwives and health visitors in the UK have the responsibility for the provision of advice and guidance to the Local Supervising Authorities (LSAs), who in turn have the responsibility for implementing the rules, requirements and guidance laid down in the statute. The English National Board describe a range of responsibilities of the supervisor, which include counselling and assisting midwives to identify their education and training needs, monitoring the practice of midwives, as well as initiating the statutory mechanism in respect of misconduct of the midwife (ENB, 1994). The supervisor must also ensure that the opportunity is provided for every midwife to meet with a supervisor at least once during the year. This, however, is an interpretation of supervision which appears much more akin to that of appraisal. In addition, in identifying these responsibilities, the question of the level of competence of the midwife being supervised is clearly raised, which in the authors' view, identifies a direct management responsibility of the supervisor. It is interpretations such as these which reflect some of the concerns practitioners have identified following the introduction of the document *A Vision for the Future*.

Mode 2: *A Vision for the Future*: the implications for clinical supervision

Although authors such as Johns (1993) demonstrate the role of clinical supervision within nursing disciplines outside those of midwifery and psychiatric nursing, it was the publication of *A Vision for the Future* that raised the concept to the top of the agenda in the context of the professional development of nursing practitioners. The document describes its function as providing a framework for the action to take account of the UKCC policy documents. The document was also developed to take forward the work of the *A Strategy for Nursing* (DoH, 1989), in particular to take account of policy initiatives in England such as *Caring for People, The Health of the Nation* and the *Patients' Charter*. The document identified twelve targets for practitioners in developing their contribution to patients' and clients' care. Target ten directly related to clinical supervision, stating that:

> discussion should be held at local and national level on the range and appropriateness of clinical supervision and a report made available to the profession by the end of the year (NHSME, 1993b, p. 15).

In defining this target the report defined clinical supervision as:

> a formal process of professional support and learning which enables professional individual practitioners to develop knowledge and competence, assume responsibility for their own practice and enhance consumer protection and the safety of care in complex clinical situations (NHSME, 1993b, p. 15).

The word competence (rather than competencies) is certainly incorporated here, and in addition this definition clearly places clinical supervision within the area of professional development rather than that of monitoring standards of care and professional conduct as outlined above in the context of midwifery supervision. The report goes on to state that clinical supervision is central to the process of learning and the expansion of the scope of professional practice of which the implications for clinical supervision are outlined below.

Indeed it is this report that has placed clinical supervision on the national agenda for the development of qualified practitioners.

Publications such as *Clinical Supervision in Practice* (Kohner, 1994) demonstrate a range of different models of clinical supervision which have occurred in response to this government initiative, but do not give more detailed guidance about how these models may be put into action, nor more importantly do they consider the expertise required of the supervisor to work effectively with the supervisee within these models. Nevertheless, both this development and the role of clinical supervision in midwifery highlight the influence of the requirements of the government and professional statutory bodies within the development of clinical supervision.

Task 1.3 Points for reflection
(alone or with a colleague)

1 Write down your own autobiography as it relates to your preparation for entry to your profession and your subsequent professional development. (Add comments about any advanced long courses that have affected your practice in the clinical setting.)

   (NB The process of writing it is important here, in order to gain maximum effect for the following tasks.)

2 Then consider the following:
   • How do your personal experiences relate to the context offered above?
   • Dig under your own written words for the origins of your own views on professional preparation and the current system, and for your own values as they relate to the preparation of practitioners and supervisors.
   • Share this with someone else and compare and contrast your own and their actual experience of preparation for practice and their emerging values.

(We all *assume* that everyone else has had the same experience and shares the same values – especially if we work together in the same practice setting or share the same professional preparation or the same qualification. The interest lies in the differences between us.)

Clinical supervision in a regulatory context

Supervision: government and professional requirements

The context in which clinical supervision takes place is also influenced by the requirements of both the government (where appropriate) and of professional bodies which speak for their professions (e.g. the Royal College of Nursing, the College of Occupational Therapy, the

Chartered Society of Physiotherapists (CSP), the British Acupuncture Council (BAcC). Since supervisors are required to operate the regulations of their profession and ought also to be contributing to discussions about future refinement and development of these, it is clearly important that they know and consider critically the relevant documents.

The following offers an overview of these issues as they relate to nursing. Colleagues in professions other than nursing will wish to consider critically their own documents, and the following task is offered to help them in doing so.

Task 1.4 Reflection for professions other than nursing

(You might wish to read the following few pages about nursing to see the kinds of thinking that are being encouraged here.)

1 What are the key regulations which relate to your work as a clinical supervisor? How have these evolved? To what extent are these national requirements and to what extent are they local (i.e. course-based or context-based)?

2 What are the key documents which publish the regulations for clinical supervision to which you have to work currently? Where have they come from, who has published them, out of what context have the documents sprung? How are they being further developed?

3 What are the overall values and assumptions on which these documents rest? What views do they hold about education and training, staff development and management?

Supervision: governmental and professional requirements in nursing

Since for nursing the responsibilities and requirements of the government in the UK vary to some extent in particular agenda according to individual country, we have selected documents which relate specifically to England in order to illustrate the implications of such policy documents to the development and context of clinical supervision. Colleagues in other parts of the UK will wish to construct and consider their own list of relevant documents.

Here, then, two major policy documents have particular implications for clinical supervision. The first of these, the National Health Service and Community Care Act 1990, made statutory the explicit requirements for the assessment of quality of care in health care provision. This demand, not only for high quality care, but also for evidence of measuring quality of care, required that practitioners assess standards of practice and make a commitment to monitoring standards and implementing change where necessary. (Such a demand, requiring the measurement of something which is essentially unmeasurable, is a key example of some of the muddled thinking currently being promoted about the work of professionals, see below p. 48). Although the *demand* for high quality care can only be applauded then, the focuses and emphasis on measurement and on standard setting raise an interesting debate for those practitioners involved in clinical supervision, particularly as the requirement to set standards does not fit easily with an approach to supervision grounded in a philosophy of reflective practice. This issue is considered in greater detail in Chapter 3.

A spin-off of this demand for quality in patient care and client care also contributed to an important document for nursing already referred to; that of a new strategy for nursing entitled *A Vision for the Future*. The aims, and the implementation, of this document as described above, have major implications for the development of clinical supervision. This is particularly so of the requirement that, following discussion at local and national level, a report should be made available to the profession on the role of clinical supervision in clinical practice. This commitment from the government led to the publication of a position paper by Faugier and Butterworth (1993). This comprehensive review of clinical supervision addressed recent literature and research, educational initiatives, examples of models of clinical supervision as well as matters relating to policy and practice. This review was circulated by the Chief Nursing Officer for England (CNO) to all directors and advisors of nursing, midwifery and health visiting within Regional Health Authorities (RHAs), District Health Authorities (DHAs), Family Health Service Authorities (FHSAs), and NHS trusts as well as to academic institutions and professional statutory bodies and organizations, 'to assist the professions in taking this important issue (clinical supervision) forward' (CNO Professional Letter, 1994). The document, in providing recommendations for taking clinical supervision forward at both a national and local level, provides a useful agenda for many of the policy issues involved in supervision. Once again, however, it gives little in the way of guidance on the processes involved in clinical supervision, or the expertise required of supervisors. Nevertheless, the commitment of the government to the concept of clinical supervision is clearly identified since the CNO stated that she had 'no doubt as to the value of clinical supervision and considered it to be fundamental to safeguarding standards, the development of professional expertise and the delivery of quality of care' (CNO Professional Letter, 1994).

In 1994 a follow-up document to the strategy for nursing was published entitled *Testing the Vision* (NHSE, 1994). In this publication a report of a survey undertaken of 609 trusts, Directly Managed Units (DMUs), RHAs, DHAs and FHSAs was provided. In an overall response rate of 52 per cent, 86 per cent of the respondents identified that they had held discussions on clinical supervision, although it should be noted that there is no evidence about the quality of such discussions. The publication also reported the circulation of the CNO's letter commending the report by Faugier and Butterworth (1993) and stating that it would provide a means of advancing discussions with members of the profession on clinical supervision.

The commitment to supervision for qualified staff by the government was demonstrated further in the CNO's letter by the commissioning of the King's Fund to produce a document to highlight the models of clinical supervision evolving within the Nursing Development Units (NDUs). This document entitled *Clinical Supervision in Practice* (Kohner, 1994) provides guidelines for the introduction and implementation of clinical supervision and examples of models in practice. The document once again, however, does not provide detailed guidance or discussion of the processes and expertise involved in supervision, although the five models of practice cover a range of professional settings in which very different practice interventions are offered and include the community, mental health and intensive care. It is interesting that in one case study, the author clearly states that the term supervision was not used, since the staff considered that the use of the term supervision threatened the practitioners' professional autonomy. Although the ten guidelines identified in the document for the implementation of clinical supervision highlight the need for all staff to be involved in the process of both planning and receiving supervision as well as the importance of appropriate preparation for practitioners taking on the role of supervisor, little guidance is offered about how this might be achieved currently within the NHS. This is particularly relevant since the final guideline identifies the need for support of the employing authority in implementing and maintaining a system of clinical supervision. The significance of this guideline for clinical supervision was demonstrated in the conference convened by the NHS Executive in November 1994, when an invited audience of over 500 nurses met to consider the implications of clinical supervision for the profession (Bishop and Butterworth, 1994; Smith, 1995).

The professional statutory bodies also have a role to play in influencing the context of clinical supervision. The regulatory body of nursing, the UKCC, in addition to the well-established professional code of conduct (UKCC, 1992b) and the document on the scope of professional practice (UKCC, 1992a), made a commitment in its 1993–1998 business plan to develop a model of clinical supervision for nurses and health visitors. This process is being undertaken in collaboration with the Department of Health in England and has been informed by the outcome of the conference described above. One important development was the publication of a position statement by the UKCC (UKCC, 1996). In this publication the Council makes a clear statement that it believes that clinical supervision will ensure the standards of professional practice by encouraging the professional development of nurses and health visitors. The Council provides six key statements which, in its view, are necessary for the effective development and practice of clinical supervision. These statements focus on issues such as the need for preparation of clinical supervisors, the requirement for the supervisee and supervisor to have a clinically-focused professional relationship and the evaluation of clinical supervision. It is noteworthy that there is no detailed reference made to the required expertise of the supervisor nor the necessary preparation for practitioners to achieve this expertise. Once more attempting to remove the association, for some professionals, with management control systems, the position statement acknowledges that clinical supervision is not to be a statutory requirement.

In addition, the recent publication by the UKCC of the proposed standards for inclusion in the contracts for hospitals and community health care services (UKCC, 1995a) also highlights the commitment of the UKCC to clinical supervision. This document recommends that in designing the content of contracts between consumers and providers of health care, mechanisms should exist to monitor the standards identified within the professional code of conduct. This includes access to clinical supervision for registered practitioners. However, by placing clinical supervision in the context of monitoring standards of practice it raises questions about the extent to which clinical supervision is seen as a monitoring exercise rather than one of professional development. This suggests a worrying degree of conflict with the philosophy of the government policy documents. Further, although the fact sheets provided on the requirements for maintaining registration discuss the concept of professional development, it is described within the context of the responsibility of the individual practitioner, rather than being seen as related to clinical supervision (UKCC, 1995b). The requirement from the statutory regulatory body for professional development remains not linked to requirements about clinical supervision.

The national boards for the education of nurses, midwives and health visitors have responsibility for the provision of advice and guidance in the implementation of the standards of practice and education determined by the UKCC. Guidelines for both the supervision of students and the practice setting in which the supervision is carried out are laid down by the English National Board (ENB). These guidelines, however, are generally written as broad principles, focusing particularly on strategies to assess the statutory learning outcomes rather than the process of student supervision. In addition, although the Board currently has no guidelines for the supervision of qualified staff, work is being undertaken collaboratively with other statutory bodies such as the UKCC, to develop and publish guidelines for the preparation of staff for the role of clinical supervisor.

Professional organizations may also play a part in influencing the context of clinical supervision. An example is provided by the Health Visitors Association (HVA), which has not only published documents about supervision but also run a national conference organized jointly with the Queen's Nursing Institute. At the conference the Chief Nursing Officer for England once again outlined the Department of Health's commitment to supervision. This commitment was reinforced by the reference to the funding by the Department of 18 sites to evaluate models of clinical supervision. The publications by the HVA include a briefing paper giving practitioners guidance on general principles and essential requirements for supervision (HVA, 1995), as well as a more detailed publication which provides models of clinical supervision and guidelines for what is described as 'training' for supervisors (Swain, 1995). This later publication, in developing the ideas of the initial briefing paper in much greater detail, sets out to describe the principles and processes of supervision. Although it provides a very clear review of the development of supervision and the different models of supervision there is little discussion of the required expertise of the supervisor in undertaking effective supervision. Once again little guidance is provided in actually carrying out supervision.

The significance of the relationship between the supervisor and supervisee is emphasized in the literature and policy documents emerging from both government and professional bodies and the emphasis on the preparation and roles and responsibilities of supervisors is clear. But the detailed matters to which supervisors need to attend have generated little debate. Yet supervisors will need to know their own strengths, recognize their uncertainties, and be able to debate new ways forward from a thought-through position but with an open mind. Interestingly then, by definition, a *training* for supervisors would not provide the basis for fulfilling such responsibilities. That which makes for quality in both of these areas, being valued-based, is complex and essentially contestable, and needs extensive and systematic exploration in educational terms. By the end of this book readers should be in a far better position to determine what makes for quality supervision. But it is thus already possible to argue that what is required to prepare supervisors for their work is education rather than training.

Clinical supervision as education

Developing a personal agenda

A careful consideration of where one starts from as a supervisor is an important basis from which to construct a personal agenda which should be of use while readers work through the rest of this book and as they seek to develop their own professional practice.

Task 1.5 Points for reflection
(alone or with a colleague)

1 Write about your own experience of supervising students (or practitioners in post) and of relating in any other way either to the preparation of students to become members of a profession or to staff development through supervision. Looking at these carefully (perhaps sharing them with a colleague) what do you learn about yourself as a supervisor?
2 What are your views about learning in the clinical setting? What role do you think the clinical supervisor should play in professional preparation or professional development?
3 Find out about the past history of supervising students and qualified practitioners in your practice setting over, say, the last 6 years. Explore these in detail. (Talk to colleagues who were involved, probe their assessment of the experience , their values, the bases of their statements).

We write in the belief that awareness of what one does and does not already know is a better base to proceed from than are assumptions. The following list is offered as an aid to clarifying both what is involved in supervision and what individual supervisors may need in order to gain new competence. Supervision education might include at least the following:

• consideration of the expertise of and possible roles for the a supervisor
• consideration of the rights and responsibilities of a supervisor
• knowledge of government and statutory requirements
• issues in the relationship of theory and practice

- practice in articulating and consideration of the principles of (theory underlying) teaching/learning
- practice in and consideration of methods of devising strategies to support the student's or practitioner's personal and professional development
- practice in observing (and in considering those observations of) students' practical work, and in understanding how this might relate to the observation and supervision of qualified staff
- practice in and consideration of a range of approaches for responding to observed practice (reflection/enabling student or practitioner to theorize/feedback/critique)
- practice in and consideration of assessing student competence in practice
- practice in and consideration of assessing need for professional development and drawing up recommendations for future training
- practice in and consideration of developing relevant interpersonal skills
- detailed knowledge about the preparation of student practitioners
- issues about what constitutes professional knowledge and educational understanding beyond practice skills
- issues relating to the student and the practice organization
- issues relating to students and professionalism
- issues in quality control, including evaluation of the practice setting.

You may wish to add other items.

To some extent much of the rest of this book is an attempt to begin to come to grips with these matters. Since what is offered here is quality supervision based upon supervisor education, the following two chapters focus upon further important issues as a basis for the more practical elements which appear later in the book. Before turning to these however, it is important to construct an agenda of your own in order to

---

Task 1.6 Points for action
(alone or with a colleague)

1 List any things that you would like to learn more about in relation to the role of professional and government bodies in clinical supervision. Consider how you might gain this information.
2 In the light of this chapter (particularly the list above) and your own reflections, list personal targets for learning to be a supervisor.*

* This list may be of interest to you again later. You may wish to review and/or refine it as you proceed through the book. You may wish to return to it at the end.

come to grips personally with what is offered and to know what you seek particularly from the following pages. Task 1.6 is an attempt to help you in this.

Further reading

Freidson, E. (1994). *Professionalism Reborn: Theory, Prophesy and Policy*. Polity Press in association with Blackwell. Ch. 12.

Hoyle, E. (1974). Professionality, professionalism and the control of teaching. *London Educational Review*, **3**, 13–18.

Langford, G. (1978). *Teaching as a Profession: an Essay in the Philosophy of Education*. Macmillan.

Colleagues should also seek for documentation on the history of their own profession.

2

Quality in professional practice: considering professionalism

Introduction

The extent to which health care professions can be considered to be *professions* remains open to debate. Authors such as Bernard and Walsh (1990), in writing about nursing for example, suggest that in part this debate rests on the definition of a profession. In offering a critique of Flexner's classical definition, which identifies six criteria including the need for the activities of the group to be intellectual, teachable and altruistic, they comment on the difficulties not only of practitioners fulfilling these criteria consistently through practice, but also of fulfilling the continuing addition of criteria to this already complex concept. Evans (1991) suggests that the debate has been furthered by the current focus on critical issues in nursing practice such as ethics, autonomy, advocacy and accountability.

Many health care professions seek various ways to emphasize their professional nature and assure the public of their own proper self-regulation. For example, like all professional bodies in health care, the role of the regulatory body for nursing, (the UKCC), emphasizes professionalism in providing a code of professional conduct which practitioners are required to maintain (UKCC, 1992b), just as the COT, the professional body for occupational therapy, provides recommendations, guidelines and directives for OTs including, for example, their *Recommended Requirements for the Accreditation of Fieldwork Educators* (COT, 1994).

There is also much published evidence that professionals themselves seek to extend their professional knowledge. For example the work of the General Council and Register of Osteopathy, in devising competencies for this new profession, was graphically shared in a recent article (Fielding and Sharp, 1995); work in acupuncture is reported regularly in, for example, the *European Journal of Oriental Medicine*, whose January 1996 issue was devoted to professional education; and that in occupational therapy which is reported in the *British Journal of*

Occupational Therapy, whose June 1995 issue was devoted to field-work education.

In addition, the public and consumers have their own expectations of the professional practice offered by health care professionals. And in all this, the growth of clinical supervision has emerged as a response to the growing demands of the professionalization of health care professions because it is generally understood that clinical supervisors contribute to maintaining professional standards within the profession.

Beneath the slippery words 'profession' and 'professional', then, lie a number of complexities about which supervisors need to be clear. Indeed, without a clear grasp of differing models of professionalism, and a thought-through position on their own preferred approach, supervisors' work with practitioners is likely to lack appropriate direction and they may experience difficulty in discussing their approach with those responsible for monitoring the quality of clinical supervision.

Clinical supervisors thus need to be familiar with the issues and debates associated with professionalism and what it is to be a member of a profession for at least four major reasons:

1 In helping practitioners develop professional practice, supervisors are engaged in professional education, and need to be clear what this enterprise involves.
2 Discussions between a supervisor and a practitioner are almost always bound to touch on issues about the role of professionals, professionalism, and practice. Even if they are not the main topic they may underlie it.
3 Since professions generally receive considerable attack in the media, practitioners, as a direct part of their continuing education, need to address the notion of professionalism and need to be prepared to discuss it with colleagues, consumers and managers.
4 Most importantly, views about professionalism (what it is to be a professional, what professionals should know and do, and how professionals think and behave) determine the kind of supervision supervisors offer to practitioners, and it is important to be aware of this, make a rational choice about it and be able to defend that choice.

What is a profession? What is professionalism?

A profession is a body of practitioners who offer public service for the public good, rather than working with products for their own profit. This indicates clearly that there is a strong moral dimension to professionalism. To be a professional is to have expert know-how underpinned by theoretical knowledge at graduate or graduate-equivalent level. The 'goods' emanating from this knowledge and accruing to individual clients must be distributed fairly and disinterestedly. Becoming a member of a profession is achieved by being approved and accepted (given professional status) as a result of assessments in both practical and theoretical dimensions of knowledge by those who are already members of the body. That approval traditionally rests not on a demonstration of mastery as a result of training but on evidence of the ability to think critically and to exercise professional judgement as a result of education. Such a professional must maintain personal standards of theoretical and practical knowledge, discipline and ethical behaviour (although there is also usually an overseeing professional council which broadly ensures standards). Professional practitioners must operate effectively and conduct themselves appropriately according to the purposes and procedures that are traditional to the profession. Central to these traditions is the (currently unfashionable) concept of service. Professionals are thus autonomous operators, in that within professional parameters they must, during practice, make considerable numbers of their own decisions using personal judgement. There is a moral dimension to this decision-making precisely because the professional's goal is to offer public service for public good.

Schön, writing from an American context, argues that the status of all professions is being eroded (see Schön, 1983, 1987). He puts this down to the fact that professions had a contract with society that in return for reliable public service they were granted autonomy, self-regulation and a certain amount of secrecy. But they have lost their status and contract because in this age of consumerism, and its resulting accountability, and at a time when authority is questioned everywhere, some professionals have been shown to make major mistakes and to have let their clients down. He evidences the many legal cases in America. These have caused society to call for the withdrawal of professional privileges, and perhaps to accord a different and much looser meaning to the word professional. Certainly Goodyear makes the point that:

> the meaning of 'professional' has slid away from the rich suggestiveness of, say, 'professional judgement', or 'professional integrity' towards the narrower end of its continuum, where it is synonymous with 'proficient', as in 'they made a very professional job of it' (Goodyear, 1992, p. 396).

Nevertheless, there are still enterprises that are generally recognized as professional. Significant examples are law and medicine. It is, however, a matter of dispute as to whether health care professions are professions of the same kind as these (see Langford, 1978). For example, although nursing has its own regulatory body which is responsible for admitting and removing practitioners from its professional register, it remains questionable whether nursing is as self-regulating and autonomous as medicine and law. Indeed the introduction of evidence of continuing study to maintain professional registration demonstrates a lack of self-regulation since central government was significant in determining whether the individual practitioners or the employer should be responsible for the provision of this continuing study. Evidence such as this may raise questions as to the extent to which nursing is *regarded* as a profession, by practitioners within the profession as well as the general public. It is, of course, in the name of protecting the public interest that professions must have careful control over preparation for entry to the profession (by means of restricted selection, clear and agreed levels of basic competence, a length of training that indicates the complexity of professional work, a clear code of ethics which is taught, major assessment of key areas of the course before registration, induction into life-long commitment to and interest in the job, and an intelligent interest in continuing professional development).

One important mark of a profession is generally acknowledged to be the need to be aware of and to grapple with complex human issues as part of practice and, at the level of the important moral dimension, there is much that can be said very clearly about health care practitioners being professionals. For example, they are clearly responsible for the distribution of important benefits, they seek to improve others, they are involved in autonomous rational judgements, they must demonstrate professional ethics, and they must work *with* rather than *on* their clients and patients in order to provide high quality care. Indeed the concept of care provides nursing with an important basis from which to demonstrate professional practice, particularly as interpretations of care become more complex and extend away from the traditional interpretation (Dalley, 1993). In addition Bruni (1991) suggests that the adoption of health promotion and rehabilitation as significant areas of nursing practice demonstrate the role that continuing development of expertise and autonomy play in professionals' practice.

It is possible, following Hoyle, to distinguish between extended and restricted professionals. He suggests in a seminal article about teachers that, unlike restricted professionals, who place value on pure experience in isolation from both broad understanding of education and also from colleagues, extended professionals are those who seek to understand their practice by considering theory and seeking broader contexts. They see classroom events in relation to social policies and goals. They share methods and ideas with colleagues, and value collaboration. They value the opportunity to be creative rather than use teacher-proofed packages. They read professional literature, are involved in in-service education and staff development, and see teaching as a thoughtful rather than a routine activity (see Hoyle, 1974).

Various authors since Hoyle have offered further sophistications to the characteristics of the extended professional, particularly in respect of being someone who investigates their own professional practice (Stenhouse, 1975), and being a reflective professional (based on the original work of Schön, 1983).

What is professional knowledge?

Pressures arising from accountability to 'state everything' about public services have led to attempts among some professional groups to list comprehensively all aspects of professional knowledge and to use that list to judge those entering the profession. But such lists are misleading. The whole point about professionalism is that it is not possible to set down simply a generally agreed detailed statement about a professional's knowledge-base. The essentially human and unique character of interaction between a professional and clients makes the detailed knowledge needed in each interaction unpredictable. A professional needs to be able to operate professional judgement and select or even create knowledge necessary to the unique situation. Practitioners need to be prepared for these processes not only through their initial preparation but also through continuing in-service education. It is also important to note that professional knowledge is far from static, but that it changes rapidly as new discoveries are made. These discoveries are either the fruits of research or of investigations by practitioners themselves. Such new knowledge is seen as an important part of practitioners' practice, not as something offered to practitioners by outside researchers. Thus, research activity and professionals' investigations and their resulting knowledge are important cutting edges for devel-

---

Task 2.1 Points for reflection
(alone or with a colleague)

1 Is your occupation a profession? What are your views so far about professionalism?
2 On what sort of occasions, in what contexts and why, do you yourself use the word professional? What do you normally mean by it?
3 Do you think Hoyle's models of extended and restricted professionals are appropriate to your profession?
4 How would you describe the key characteristics of your own professionalism?

oping professional practice. The whole issue of professionalism and preparation for becoming a professional is thus highly complex and to try to simplify it is to distort it (Task 2.1).

So, from the above discussion it is possible to see the complexities involved in clinical supervision, professional practice and continuing professional development. The following is an attempt to demonstrate these issues in more detail. It provides a rationale for the rest of this book and a challenge to all who are involved in clinical supervision to consider their own stance towards being a professional and supervising others within the profession.

Two models of professional practice explored

Some people, then, see the initial preparation of practitioners as offering would-be professionals a set of clear-cut routines and behaviours and a pre-packaged content which requires only an efficient means of delivery. This cuts down considerably, they argue, the risks that professionals might fail to provide a reliable service. This in turn makes assumptions that practice is a relatively simple interaction in which the practitioner gives and patients and clients receive. Others, however, feel that this denies the real character of both professionalism on the one hand and practice on the other. They argue that professional practice involves complex decision-making and elements of professional judgement and practical wisdom guided by moral principles but that these are not able to be set down in absolute routines.

One view of professionalism characterizes professional activities as essentially simple, describable and able to be broken down into their component parts (skills) and thus mastered. It regards being a professional as being essentially efficient in skills, and submissive in harnessing them to carry out other people's decisions. An example in nursing is perhaps provided by the introduction of National Vocational Qualifications (NVQ). This scheme has been described as a new approach to training provided at five different levels, determined by units of competence. Indeed it is suggested that this approach provides students with a clearly-defined set of competencies in a specific area of practice. Although designed for a range of academic ability, level five is described as being equivalent to a higher degree or final year undergraduate work (Mangan, 1995). Similar approaches to thinking about practice have been adopted in other professions too, like occupational therapy, physiotherapy and osteopathy. In some cases the term 'performance outcomes' replaces 'competencies', but they are essentially the same. Indeed, Fielding and Sharp (1995) provide details of the work carried out in osteopathy to produce seven levels, 50 elements and 240 components of osteopathy which make up the list of competencies to practice. The idea that practitioners are accountable for a set of competencies within a defined area of practice, however, suggests they are answerable only for the technical accuracy of their work within the bounds of achieving other people's goals. In other words, the professional's role becomes purely instrumental, and even, arguably, is reduced below the level of what can be called professional. This is the technical–rational view of professional practice. It has at its base what Raymond Williams described as the industrial trainers' approach to education (Williams, 1965).

It can be seen as diametrically opposed to the view in which behaving professionally is seen as being concerned with both means and ends. Here, professional activity is more akin to artistry, and practitioners are broadly autonomous, making their own decisions about their actions and the moral bases of those actions. In this model the professional is not less accountable, but is in fact accountable for more. Here, to be professional is to be morally accountable for all of one's conduct. Here the ability to exercise professional judgement is seen as essential and professional judgement is not a simple skill. In fact this view of professional practice rejects the notion that it can be divided into simple skills. It considers that professional activity includes components which cannot be entirely disentangled and treated separately. It takes a more holistic view. This has been called the professional artistry view (see Schön, 1987). The influence of this view can be seen particularly in the important work of Mattingly and Fleming (1994) in occupational therapy and the interest in clinical reasoning that it has sparked off in that and allied professions (see, especially Higgs and Jones, 1995). Yet professional artistry is generally less well documented, partly because the climate has been against it even though it is very much alive in some professionals' practice. In nursing, even recent literature makes little use of the term (see, for example, Palmer, Burns and Bulman, 1994), but reflections on nursing actions published by practitioners such as L'Aiguille (1994) provide clear evidence that interest in it is developing.

In all of this, then, questions are raised about what professional expertise should consist of and therefore what professionals should do in order to learn and then to continue to develop their practice.

Some would argue that professional practice has for too long been surrounded by a mystique and has now advanced to the point where goals can be set by society for professionals whose role is purely instrumental. For example they might point to the very language of health care today, including 'clinical guidelines; clinical outcomes; health outcome indicators; health technology assessment; all form part of NHS strategies for improving the effectiveness of the service it provides' (Culshaw, 1995, p. 223). They would argue that the professional's role can now be analysed technically and rationally in terms of activities and skills (the professional craft knowledge) (see Alsop, 1993), and that all that remains is to teach these to the professional trainee. Here, to learn professional practice is to identify and then to practise skills until they have been mastered, and then to learn to apply them with success to real situations. The language is not about professional *competence* (an holistic concept) but of individual *competencies* (an atomizing of skills). To improve practice is to move on to harder skills and more complex situations. This offers an incremental view of practice. The fact that many of these competencies are simple and can be quickly taught, simply practised and easily measured or observed is also regarded as entirely desirable in a world of diminishing resources.

By contrast, however, some would argue that the technical–rational view of professionalism which offers simple pre-set routines and procedures, skills and knowledge, does not meet the real situations of practice. They would emphasize the idea that practice is messy, unpredictable, unexpected, and requires the ability to improvise (an ability often *diminished* by training and routine). In short it requires professional artistry, well beyond technical efficiency, or routine craft skills. Also, practice is rapidly changing and requires the practitioner autonomously to be able to refine and update his or her expertise 'on the hoof'. The problem seen with the technical–rational approach to professional practice is that it simply leads in the end to an obsessive intention to tie things down further and further in the inevitably vain attempt to try to cater for all eventualities. Here, by contrast, to prepare for successful professional practice is to be educated roundly, not drilled in skills. To improve practice is to treat it more holistically, to work to understand its complexities, and to look carefully at one's actions and theories as one works and, subsequently, to challenge them with ideas from other perspectives, and to seek to improve and refine practice and its underlying theory. Here the professional is working towards increased competence. Some would argue that this is all too woolly (because it admits of less certainty). Further, it does not please politicians because its fruits may show up less clearly in the short term since it emphasizes aspects that are not simple, visible behaviours. But, in the long term, it offers scope for deeper rooted improvements, which are owned by the professional.

Thus, the technical–rational (TR) view believes in the centrality of rules, schedules, prescriptions, whereas the professional artistry (PA) view believes that practice starts where the rules fade (because the rules rarely fit real practice). Thus, the PA view relies on frameworks and rules of thumb, rather than rules. The TR view emphasizes diagnosis, analysis, and efficient systems. It believes in detailed job specifications and in being able to analyse a professional role down to the last detail.

The PA view by contrast, believes instead in interpretation of details, acknowledges the inevitable subjectivity of setting them down, and comes to an understanding of professional activities by means of appreciation (as in the critical appreciation of art and music). It wishes to encourage not narrow efficiency but creativity and the right to be wrong. The TR model assumes that knowledge is permanent, able to be totally mastered, and thus worth attempting to master. The PA view is that knowledge is temporary, dynamic and problematic, and that knowing processes is more useful than knowing facts.

Their impact on practice and theory

But it is, perhaps, in its views about theory that the TR model is most highly specific. It sees theory as 'formal theory' produced by researchers (who stand apart from the practitioners). This formal theory is to be learnt and then applied to practice. It regards practice as an arena in which to demonstrate previously worked-out theory. This makes for problems when practice becomes more complex and human in its demands. Mattingly and Fleming illustrate the impact of this on health care professionals in OT as follows:

> The model of professional reasoning treated as applied science presumes that the work of the practitioner is simply to identify which means (including techniques) will best get one to the ends required; hence such thinking is often referred to as *means-ends rationality or technical rationality*. The end, the final goal . . . is not what scientific reasoning is designed to consider.

They add that when the goal becomes questionable as in a dying patient on a life support system:

> this is marginalized in the medical profession as a problem of ethics, which is distinguished from a problem of clinical decision making (Mattingly and Fleming, 1994, p. 11).

This view, that theory is formal and applicatory, has also affected professional education. It has led in the past to the old traditional approach to course design in which blocks of theory were followed by periods of practice in order to 'apply' the knowledge in the practice situation. By contrast, the PA view is that theory is implicit in (underlies) all action, that both action and theory are developed in practice, that refining practice involves unearthing the theories on which it is founded and that formal theory aids the development of practice by challenging and extending the practitioner's understandings. This view, that (with the help of reflection) theory emerges *from* practice, enables the professional training course to begin with *practice*, and to enable the student to examine and develop personal theory as it arises from that practice. Such personal theory is implicit in all action but needs to be exhumed from it in order to be acknowledged, understood, and used to inform decisions about later action. It is also able to be refined by recourse to further practice and to the wider view of theory offered by other theorists and researchers. Chapters 3, 4 and 6 illustrate this in much more detail and provide practical assistance for supervisors in considering their own practice and helping practitioners to do the same.

Their views of professional activities

There are other characteristics that distinguish the two different views of professionalism enshrined in these models. These consist of views about and attitudes towards professional activity. For example, the technical–rational view believes in the mastery of skills and knowledge, and regards becoming a professional as acquiring sets of competencies. These can be taught by training. The technical–rational view, then, emphasizes the 'known', and is in tune with present trends in that it celebrates certainty and hard evidence as opposed to uncertainty, humility and critical scepticism. Professional practice in this model is made up from a series of definable skills, measurable by means of observation, and influenced by researchers who are called in from another world.

By contrast the professional artistry view is willing to accept the notion of mystery within human activity. It regards the activity of the professional as not entirely able to be analysed down to the last atom even if the routinized craft skills on which artistry is based are able to be specified. It regards professional practitioners as eternal seekers rather than 'knowers'. It sees the activities of the professional as mainly open capacities which by definition are not able to be mastered. The test of an open capacity is that the learner can take steps which he has not been taught to take, which in some measure surprise the teacher, that he can 'do the unexpected, . . . do it well, efficiently and at the right time' (Passmore, 1980, pp. 42–3). The professional artistry view, then, sees professional practice as an art in which risks are inevitable, learning to do is only achieved by engaging in doing, together with reflecting upon the doing, and where improvization, enquiry into action and resulting insight by those involved in it generate a major knowledge-base.

Their differing views of quality

Each model gives rise to a particular view of quality. The technical–rational model speaks in the language of quality control. It places emphasis upon visible performance within the practical aspects of the course. It seeks to test and measure these, believing that technical expertise is all-important and that learning cashes out immediately into visible products. Thus the model is behaviourist, emphasizes fixed standards, controls the course via inspection and appraisal, and believes that change can be imposed from outside the profession and that quality is measurable. It wishes to hold the professional practitioner accountable only for his or her technical expertise.

By contrast, the professional artistry view sees that there is more to professional practice than its surface and visible features. It believes that there is more to the whole than the sum of the parts, it believes in professional judgements, and holds that the most easily measurable is often also the most trivial. Further, it wishes to harness investigation, reflection and deliberation in order to enable professionals to develop their own insights from inside and holds that this is a better means of staff development than innovation imposed from without. In short, it believes that quality comes from deepening insight into one's own values, priorities, actions. Under this model it is possible to talk about wide professional answerability rather than narrow technical accountability. This introduces not only a responsibility for the moral dimensions of professional action, but also the responsibility to reflect upon, investigate and refine one's own practice.

Table 2.1 offers a summary of the points above.

To look closely at these two very different views of professionalism is to recognize among their views some clear incompatibilities. Some argue that these views are extreme versions of a continuum along which individuals can find their own place. Others hold them to be ultimately antithetical, requiring harder decisions to be made about where one stands. But we would wish to point out that these two views are not two of a kind as might be suggested by presenting them in parallel (which we do only in order to emphasize the contrast between them). In fact the TR view is a closed-system view of practice in that it is concerned exclusively with skills as ends in themselves and believes in the possibility of analysing these in absolute detail, and that all that matters is mastering them. By contrast, the PA view does not exclude skills but rather focuses on providing professionals with an educated understanding out of which the professional can then select skills appropriate to context and learn to operate and develop them in practice.

It is important, then, for supervisors to consider these positions carefully because the models themselves give rise to two distinct

Table 2.1 Two views of professional practice

The technical–rational view	*The professional artistry view*
Follows rules, laws, schedules	Starts where rules fade
Uses routines, prescriptions	Sees patterns, frameworks
Uses diagnosis, analysis to think about professional practice	Uses interpretation and appreciation to think about professional practice
Wants efficient systems	Wants creativity and room to be wrong
Sees knowledge as graspable, permanent	Sees knowledge as temporary, dynamic, problematic
Theory is applied to practice	Theory emerges from practice
Visible performance is central	There is more to it than surface features
Setting out and testing for basic competence is vital	There is more to professional practice than the sum of the parts
Technical expertise is all	Professional judgement counts
Sees professional activities as masterable	Sees mystery at the heart of professional activities
Emphasizes the known	Embraces uncertainty
Standards must be fixed Standards are measurable Standards must be controlled	That which is most easily fixed and measurable might also be trivial – professionals should be trusted
Emphasizes assessment, appraisal, inspection, accreditation	Emphasizes investigation, reflection, deliberation
Change must be managed from outside	Professionals can develop from inside
Quality is really about quantity of that which is easily measurable	Quality comes from deepening insight into one's values, priorities, actions
Technical accountability	Professional answerability
This is training	This is education
It takes the instrumental view of learning	It sees education as intrinsically worthwhile

approaches to the preparation of practitioners. It is these approaches which in turn colour and shape practice in the clinical setting. To work as a supervisor with practitioners is to take a stand on these matters – whether consciously or not. Professions too are becoming more aware of these models, as the preparation for a whole range of practitioners becomes rooted in philosophies developed collaboratively with higher education. Supervisors, then, may find it impossible to offer a rationale for their practice and to cope with practitioner queries about practice without recourse to these issues and a clear idea of their own views about them. Quality supervision certainly demands no less.

Task 2.2 Points for reflection

Models are dangerous in their simplification and polarizing of issues. This is because they are reductionist. That is, they reduce matters to crude elements that do not do justice to the complexities found in practice. They are useful only if, by highlighting and emphasizing differences, they enable issues to be considered which will then enlighten practice. What are your views so far about the models presented in this chapter?

Two models of clinical supervision

As indicated in Chapter 1, there appear to have been two major influences on the development of clinical supervision of qualified practitioners in nursing, and these provide examples of how differing approaches to clinical supervision can develop. One influence on clinical supervision in nursing has come from the disciplines of psychotherapy and counselling as seen in psychiatric nursing, while the second, the ongoing assessment of competence, has been developed in midwifery supervision. These influences have created the development of two distinct approaches to clinical supervision. The first of these is an eclectic approach, but one which has focused on reflection and the development of understanding and self-awareness in the practitioner. The second approach places an emphasis on the required skills for competence in practice as demonstrated by the approach used in midwifery practice. The resulting two distinct views of supervision are the reflective practitioner philosophy and that of competency-based supervision. Due to the developmental stage of clinical supervision in nursing practice, it seems that supervisors have a tendency to adopt parts of both these models, adding to the confusion of the role of clinical supervision in practice. Indeed this causes a number of tensions, since for some people at least, the two approaches are incompatible. At best they do not sit easily together, having opposing views about the basic nature of the task of supervising professional practitioners. There is a serious issue here for professions still developing their approach to clinical supervision. The details of the differing approaches are now offered below.

Competency-based clinical supervision

At root, competency-based supervision treats practice as if it were an occupation rather than a profession. Here professional practice is seen in terms of a set of competencies. These are not simply of prime importance, but are the *only* important focus. Theory (of any kind) is not regarded as important. What is considered most important in this approach is mastering specific and standardized skills and demonstrating that mastery. The skills are thus turned into competencies and used as the means of assessing performance in the clinical area. Such an approach, though useful in factory production, where there is only one right way of doing things and where professional judgement is irrelevant, is incompatible with professional activity. Indeed, dividing professional practice into collections of skills which can be seen and measured distorts the nature of practice, not only because there is much more to being a practitioner than that, but also because there is unlikely to be universal agreement about exactly how many skills are necessary. For example:

- How and from where will such skills be derived? (On what base model of practice will they be chosen?)
- How explicitly and in what detail should they be defined?
- How many should there be?
- What will count as evidence for their acquisition? (How many times must they be demonstrated before they are deemed to be acquired?)
- Will practitioners need to be competent in them all, and should they strive to be practised in each at the same level?
- What order of priority will they be given, and how?
- How will experience affect the level expected? (Should beginning practitioners have to demonstrate less than the full range, and if so which should be left till later?)

The arguments for competency-based approaches to clinical supervision arise in part from a bureaucratic approach which wishes to control professions by measuring the quality of care, and determining in specific terms what constitutes safe professional practice. In part it also stems from the belief that advantages accrue from using competencies to establish a large amount of uniformity within (and even striving for it across) professions (see, for example, Fielding and Sharp, 1995). Harvey, Mason and Ward (1995) argue that professional statutory bodies should come together on a broad scale with higher education providers and define the specific competencies together with their underpinning knowledge that are needed to become an effective professional practitioner. They talk of explicit skills and 'knowledge templates', and threshold standards of attainment, and an indication of the current concern about competence and competencies can be seen in the publication in *Complementary Therapies in Medicine* (volume 3, number 1, January 1995) of an issue which is devoted to considering competence and validation across health care professions.

Competency-based approaches to professional practice are processes in which it is thought that it is possible to observe and measure a set of skills, for which the supervisor and practitioner are accountable. This approach has perhaps arisen, in part, because of the muddling of 'competence' (a broad ability, which surely no one would wish to disown as part of professionalism), with the quite different notion of 'competencies' or 'competency' (individual skills which can be identified by analysing professional practice down to its last sub-skill). The work of David Carr shows that the first of these, 'competence', is the wider and more holistic, and is understood in the *capacity* sense (capacities entail 'the voluntary and deliberate exercise of principled judgement [about when and how to deploy skills] in the light of rational knowledge and understanding' (Carr, 1993, p. 257)). It is the result of education. The second, 'competency' is narrower, more atomistic and could be understood in the *dispositional* sense. (Learning dispositions means learning skills and habits on the assumption that they will be employed *as learnt*.) This requires only training in skills.

In summary, it could be said, then, that competence will be striven for by an educated practitioner who is free to make professional judgements in the practical context according to his or her reading of that situation, whereas competencies can enslave the practitioner who has been trained to operate pre-learnt skills in the practical situation without a prior and detailed reading of that context, and who has become not an autonomous professional, but merely a puppet of others.

Carr shows that it is easy to relate and confuse the two ('competence' and 'competency') particularly when the singular ('competence') is wrongly used as a dispositional term. In fact, a *skill*, should be referred to as a 'competency' and not as a 'competence'. Competency, when pluralized, follows the normal grammatical rule, changing 'y' for 'ies'. Thus the plural of 'competency' is 'competencies'. There is, technically, no such thing as 'competences' since the word 'competence' already refers to a holistic *range* of attributes and would have no plural version.

In the supervision of clinical practice, it is vital to hold competence and competency apart. Clearly there is a world of difference between thinking about behaviour resulting from an educated understanding (competence) on the one hand and professional practice in terms of pre-specifiable, discrete, itemized skills (competencies) on the other. It is a distinction, as Carr says between, on the one hand, working: 'in a broadly principled, reflective and informed way', and on the other, putting learnt routines into efficient operation (see Carr, 1993, p. 262). Knowledge of principles enables professionals to adapt and improvise, whatever the situation, whereas trained operators simply follow routines. The problem for the trained operator, is that when the learnt routines no longer fit the situation there might be total breakdown, not simply some loss of efficiency, and such situations occur often for professionals who work with people. This makes training more suitable for conveyor-belt operators who work with objects, than for professionals who work with clients.

Although of course, technical questions about efficiency are always important, a key problem for the clinical supervisor arises because such emphasis is currently placed on visible performance in assessing students or working in professional development with colleagues. For example, it is possible for a reflective practitioner to perform badly in terms of dispositional effectiveness, and for his or her important attributes (like recognition of practical shortcomings and understanding about how to improve future practice) to be ignored. On the other hand, it is also possible for an effective practitioner to perform routinely well but without any principled understanding. The key issue here is how these two types of practitioner might be improved and, whereas the former might fairly easily and quickly be helped by practising some skills in the practical setting, the latter would need to gain extensive educational understanding before knowing how to improve practice. As Carr concludes:

> professional competence in the capacity sense cannot be reduced to a set of competencies in the dispositional sense. . . . (Carr, 1993, p. 264).

Thus there are greater problems in improving practice when only skills have been learnt as routines (in a competency-based course) than when the professional has been educated and can think at the level of principle.

In summary we would wish to argue, then, that the creation of lists of competencies and the view that they provide unproblematic objectives for clinical supervision and a simple means of assessing professional practice are an attempt to:

- introduce a simple skills-based approach to professional practice
- substitute the notion of competencies for the notion of competence

and thus reduce the status and significance of professionalism
- simplify the problematic (as if practice is merely a matter of learning a few skills and strategies)
- make 'plain sense' out of the genuinely complex (as if the skills and strategies sought are straightforward and are known and agreed by everyone)
- present knowledge as absolute when much is still unknown
- de-politicize the essentially political (as if matters beyond acquiring and using the basic skills and knowledge set out are not the business of practitioners)
- render amoral the deeply m28oral (as if there are no issues at stake beneath these skills about what is – and what is not – offered to patients and clients by practitioners)
- universalize the eternally contestable (as if practice skills and strategies are not only agreed by everyone but are applicable in every situation)
- pretend the possibility of objectivity in the face of certain subjectivity (as if, because the competencies are now set out and clearly determined, there remains no subjectivity in the process of supervision).

The creation of lists of competencies appears to offer simple measures of efficiency. Yet such apparently sure foundations are easily revealed as false. However, within the Health Service at the current time the emphasis is clearly placed on value for money and the cost effectiveness of services. Within this context supervisors need to understand the role that competencies play in supervision and consider their use in professional development. Chapter 7 focuses upon this in great detail, providing a range of practical possibilities (Task 2.3).

Although competencies may reflect the current context and philosophy of the management structure of the National Health Service, many practitioners subscribe to at least some of the elements of the other main approach, which is discussed below.

Reflective practitioner philosophy

The arguments for taking a reflective practitioner approach to clinical supervision are derived from the professional artistry view of practice. Broadly the arguments are as follows.

The world of professional practice is fast changing. Professionals need to exercise and to continue to refine and develop not only simple skills, but their own dispositions, personality/professional character, abilities, capacities, understandings. Many aspects of practice cannot be

---

Task 2.3 Points for action and reflection

1 Think about the competencies required for your particular area of practice:
   - identify those which are most appropriate to assess the quality of practice
   - what else is important to consider in assessing a practitioner's competence?
2 Under what circumstances might competencies accentuate performance at the expense of understanding?
3 Is it reasonable to label knowledge, values, attitudes and personal attributes as competencies?
4 Where, in competency-based training, does the practitioner's motivation come from?
5 List the competencies that supervisors might be asked to master. Then compare your list with the list on pages 31–32 above, and your own personal agenda produced at the end of Chapter 1. Make a note about what you discover.

---

pre-specified. Professionals need to be able to think on their feet, to improvise, to respond to the uncharted and unpredictable. Furthermore, health care professionals engage in moral and social practices and exercise moral decision-making and professional judgement. What is needed is an approach to practice and the supervision of practice which enables practitioners 'to work at their practice, modify it and keep it under critical control' (Eraut, 1989, p. 175). As Eraut later argues, 'both transfer to a wider range of situations and further improvement of performance in familiar situations are difficult to achieve without . . . critical consciousness of what one is doing and why'. He argues that once one becomes more aware of the nature and effect of one's own theories, then it is possible to consider those of others. Equally, in recognizing the contexts in which one's theories have been developed, one will become better able to identify the point at which new theories are necessary as new situations arise (see Eraut, 1989, p. 184).

When practitioners claim that the underlying philosophy of their practice is that of the reflective practitioner it means far more than the rather obvious point that practitioners should think about what they do as practising professionals. Rather it refers to an approach to practice in which a *systematic* process of properly structured *critical enquiry* into one's own practice is used to examine and refine that practice. Some argue that Schön's version of reflection (Schön, 1983, 1987), is inherently conservative in that it does not involve radical challenge to the practitioner's values and views, but merely expects the practitioner to oscillate between action and thought (see, for example, Ashcroft and Foreman-Peck, 1994). But this need not be so. Indeed, the term reflective practice has been coined to imply quite the opposite – that the practitioner will investigate practice and draw up to it a range of challenging perspectives from theory. For disputes about the exact meaning of this term reflective practitioner see Calderhead (1988) and (1989) and Russell (1993b). Calderhead, within the context of teaching, points to the fact that many terms exist like 'reflective practice', 'enquiry-oriented teacher education', 'teacher as researcher', 'teacher as decision-maker', 'teacher as problem-solver', and that all of these embrace the notion of reflection, but add to it a range of other and differing ideas. He also draws attention to the fact that the key theorists on whose work the notion of reflective practice is based include Dewey and Schön. He shows that reflective teaching has 'become a slogan, disguising numerous practices' (Calderhead, 1989, p. 46) and that there is as yet no clear language in which to discuss these matters.

This situation is equally pertinent to nursing. Reflective practice, then, is a developing concept, in need of further work and subject at the moment to particular pressures from an antithetical climate (see Golby, 1993b, pp. 4–9 and 41). Nevertheless, it seems to have offered a common enough set of characteristics for practitioners to identify its character as including:

- taking practice *and* personal and formal theory seriously and being aware of their complexities
- taking a holistic view of professional practice
- taking a problem-solving stance to practice
- recognizing the need for the practitioner to investigate practice personally and valuing small-scale humanistic enquiry
- seeking the 'meaning in the experience' by means of reflecting on it
- seeking to identify beneath practice the values, assumptions, beliefs and personal theories (or 'theories of action')
- working in collaboration with colleagues, the better to reflect, deliberate and understand practice
- doing all this in order to develop/change/refine/challenge practice.

Since the term reflection is central to this approach, it is also important to understand something of its nature within this context, and to try to be clear about how it relates to other similar concepts.

Reflection is one means of investigating practice and of theorizing about it. Basically it involves *systematic* critical and creative thinking about action with the intention of understanding its roots and processes and thus being in a position to refine, improve, or change future actions. It is related to, but different from evaluation, deliberation, appraisal, self-appraisal and audit. Appraisal, self-appraisal and audit, might be described as interested in the (immediate) success of the professional practitioners' *performance*. Evaluation and self-evaluation might be seen as seeking evidence which will enable practitioners to measure the results of practice against their objectives. Deliberation is described by Schwab (1969) as a process of corporate discussion about future actions based upon weighing data and professional judgements. Reflection, on the other hand, while sharing with the others a research/investigative base, and being, like them, a response to quality control issues and an aid in the attempt to improve future actions, is unlike them in that it is interested in:

- understanding the deeper and interrelated processes of the particular thought and action, rather than displaying their surface and apparently separable features
- identifying the personal theories of the practitioner and considering how they might be refined
- recognizing the values and beliefs that underlie the particular practitioner's actions.

In these respects reflection touches matters that are both more intimate and more difficult to acknowledge than are other approaches to investigating practice (like, for example, some forms of action research). Arguably also, it unearths issues that are at the very centre of understanding and refining individual practice.

There is not one but a number of ways in which practitioners can reflect upon action. Schön has pointed out that reflection can take place during the action itself (this he calls reflection-in-action) and/or it can take place after the action as a result of looking back upon it (this he calls reflection-on-action) (see Schön, 1987). Chapter 6 looks at these in detail.

This view of professional practice raises deep questions about what kind of professional expertise (professional body of knowledge) professionals need to learn, what their educators need to foster in them, and what supervisors need to observe and evaluate. Given the notion that clinical practice involves practical problem-solving where practitioners seek to understand inevitably unique situations to which they have to offer a creative response, it raises questions not only about the extent to which practitioners can be prepared for these situations, but also about the supervision of practitioners. (Clearly they cannot be *trained* for the unexpected.) However, what is involved is creating conditions for, and a means of monitoring, the development of professional artistry. What is the relevant expertise then that practitioners are trying to develop, and how can supervisors facilitate this development?

The expertise sought is practical wisdom and professional judgement. It might best be achieved by wide-ranging preparation in addition to practice in specific skills. Such preparation would aim at providing something of the following:

- appreciation of the complexities of practice and how that practice is developed
- the ability and capacity to investigate practice
- the ability and capacity to refine practice
- the ability and capacity to theorize from practice
- the ability and capacity to reflect on practice in a systematic and rigorous way
- an understanding of the complexity of the relationship between thought and action
- knowledge of formal theory and of how to harness it to enlighten practice.

In short, practitioners need to develop the *art* of the practical (ways of harnessing theory and practice) by means of practice and practical discourse. Ways have to be found of supervising this process, and providing feedback to both the successful and unsuccessful practitioner.

The rest of the chapters of this book attempt to look in detail at how supervisors can provide these conditions, and carry out supervision within this context.

Implications for supervisors

An important implication for supervisors using a competency-based approach to supervision is the need to take a behaviourist approach to their own practice and that of the practitioner. This suggests that they must be able to demonstrate that they themselves possess these skills. In addition, a major focus for their discussions with practitioners will be the required competencies for that area of practice. It would be possible to supervise practitioners on this basis with relatively little recourse to the theoretical aspects of practice. Indeed there is no need for reference to the practitioners' theories, assumptions, beliefs that underlie and inform their practice. There is no need to discuss the decision-making that has informed practice, beyond the simple technical decisions about the means adopted within the context of that particular area of practice. The culmination of such supervision is that practitioners will be able to carry out the process of self-assessment against the list of competencies given and become a self-directing technical practitioner, generally limiting the extent to which they will be able to respond effectively to the challenges of a continually changing professional environment.

The demands on supervisors adopting the reflective practice philosophy, on the other hand, are considerable. Those offering professional supervision shaped by this philosophy will need to have certain skills and adopt certain responsibilities. As a result they will also gain enormously in terms of their own professional development. However, it assumes that supervisors have the knowledge and skills to operate as reflective practitioners themselves, that they can unearth the theory beneath their practice, challenge it with ideas drawn from other perspectives, refine it and investigate the refinements. It assumes that those supervising practice will be able to work with practitioners to help them tackle the complex matters of their professional aims and will be able to encourage them to face up to their uncertainties as well as the need to reconsider their values.

The following chapters are an attempt to explore these issues in greater detail.

Task 2.4 Points for action and reflection

1 Look in detail at one episode of clinical supervision you have undertaken recently and try to decide what aspects of it drew upon professional artistry.
2 What characteristics ought a quality supervisor to have? (Why?)
3 What rationales do you think ought to be the basis of professional practice? (Why?)
4 Have you changed or extended your opinions about any of these matters as a result of your reading so far?

Further reading

Burke, J. (ed.) (1989). *Competency-based education and training*. Falmer Press. See especially Chapters 1 and 2.

Fish, D. (1989). *Learning Through Practice in Initial Teacher Training*. Kogan Page. Chapters 2–4.

Hoyle, E. (1974). Professionality, professionalism and the control of teaching. *London Educational Review*, **3**, 13–18.

Langford, G. (1978). *Teaching as a Profession: an Essay in the Philosophy of Education*. Macmillan.

Osterman, K. and Kottcamp, R. (1993). *Reflective Practice for Educators*. Corwin Press Inc.

3

Quality learning through practice: unearthing meaning from experience

Introduction: the primacy of practice and its relationship to theory

Many programmes of professional preparation for health care have until recently been based upon an applicatory view of theory and practice (where practice was the place to apply pre-learnt theory). Some of the impetus for moving beyond this view has come from linking professional preparation more closely to higher education, where more sophisticated debates about theory and practice have always taken place. For example, schools of occupational therapy began seriously to look at the relationship between theory and practice in the early 1980s as the diploma in occupational therapy was being introduced and the degree was beginning to be conceived. Further, it was only in 1986 that Project 2000 began to provide a radical new framework for nurse preparation, raising as it did so issues about the need for competent nurses to be able to build and transfer their knowledge to meet changing health needs, thus revealing the need for the profession to consider more sophisticated relationships between theory and practice (UKCC, 1986). And in some newly emerging professions, like acupuncture, the influence of the applicatory view of theory is still evident today, although curriculum development has begun apace in the colleges.

In nursing, the profession has responded to Project 2000 by attempting recently, in its preparation programmes, to integrate theory and practice on the basis of developing the 'knowledgeable doer' (someone who having understood principles, can shape their practice to respond to the changing health needs they meet, and who can also anticipate future developments in practice). It is also the case that for many decades there has been an attempt to move nursing into higher education, which was in part achieved by the early 1960s, and which now emphasizes the need to think carefully about the design and balance of pre-registration programmes and in addition how they articulate with post-registration education.

Ironically (and apparently without logic) by contrast, in the parallel field of teacher education, the public and politicians (who have had a great influence upon the shape of initial training courses for teachers) have, since the late 1980s, been going through a phase of denigrating theory, seeing it as 'something outside the practice of teaching' (Stones, 1992, p. 279). This seems to be because in favouring the importance of practice alone in producing good teachers it will ultimately be made possible to remove teacher education from higher education altogether.

Many educators revile this view. Stones, for example, who draws on vast experience of working with teachers and student teachers, shows that those who argue for the importance of practice alone, in fact see learning to teach as learning a craft skill. Here, neophyte teachers learn by observing other teachers and the procedures consist of a limited circle of trial, error and folk wisdom. As a result, this version of learning on the job is unsystematic, and unable to be generalized. Further, the teacher's role is that of passing on information to the student just as they might to pupils. And the lack of an underlying theory about teaching and learning:

> confines any discussion between experienced and beginning teachers to surface activities of teaching (Stones, 1992, p. 9).

Such a view of theory and practice is a result of a fundamental lack of basic philosophical understanding about what professional practice involves, and therefore how it might be learnt and how the learner might be assisted.

What is offered here is a book which is based upon a belief in the primacy of practice, and the importance of its underlying theory to all who work in health care professions. That is, it takes as its starting point the idea that in learning any aspect of professional practice (both learning to be a practitioner and learning to be a clinical supervisor) the professional, or student, should *begin* with action. But this is emphatically not the same as saying that learning something practical is *only* achieved by action, neither is it the same as saying that only practice is of any significance and that theory should be set on one side. Indeed, put simply, there is a closer interrelationship between theory and practice than the lay person understands. No action, unless it is the action of a madman (an irrational being), is devoid of theory, for theory involves beliefs, ideas, assumptions, values, and everything we do is thus influenced by theory. What may be absent, of course, is *awareness* of such theories. Thus to speak of training nurses only in practical things would be a nonsense.

Clearly, as a basic platform for their work, *quality* clinical supervisors need to know the philosophical arguments for their practices and to have a grasp of the traditions in which they are working. They also need to have up-to-date research knowledge about learning to become practitioners. Over the last few years considerable progress has been made in understanding how to enable students to learn to become health professionals, though by no means all is yet understood. Indeed, the excitement of working in this area is that it is an evolving field, where much is still to be learnt. This requires a knowledge of present levels of understanding as a sound base for further development, and an enjoyment of working at the edge of the unknown. It also requires a tolerance of uncertainty. Further, clinical supervisors may well find that they need to explain these ideas and procedures and discuss them with students, colleagues, clients and managers. The following pages therefore seek to look in some detail at some of the supporting philosophies, principles, processes, and traditions of learning professional practice via two major issues: what is involved in learning something practical; and what is involved in learning professional practice. Finally, by implication from these two, clinical supervisors will be asked to consider what can be said so far about how such learning might be fostered and assisted.

We believe, as Russell also argues about initial teacher training, that an attempt to come to grips with the details of how we learn through practice is a much neglected and yet vital aspect of professional education, and therefore of supervision. Talking of student teachers who are trying to discover how to learn from experience, he makes the point that because their supervisors have not:

> experienced a practicum that concentrated on learning from experience, they have no appropriate images and models to support such purposes (Russell, 1993a, p. 208).

A similar situation exists in nursing. The next section uses practical work that we often include in clinical supervisor workshops in an attempt to tackle this issue.

A practical experience and some reflections

Learning something practical

Quality supervision, then, involves a detailed understanding and appreciation of how we learn new practice and therefore how the learner can be supported in doing so. The implications of this for professional practice are set out in the second main section of this chapter. In order to gain full insight from that part of the chapter, readers will need first of all to try out a new piece of practice following the instructions in Task 3.1. Being willing to experience and investigate one's own practice (even a very simple piece of practice) is a vital base from which to work with practitioners for whom the supervisor has a responsibility. Being ready to learn, and knowing about oneself as a learner, are important bases for learning through practice and thus are important attributes of a clinical supervisor (see, for example, Higgs, 1992). Anyone not interested in working at their own practice in this way would be advised to consider carefully exactly what it is they as supervisors have to offer practitioners.

For the purpose of the rest of this chapter we take learning professional practice as a version of practical problem-solving – i.e. as an activity in which one can make progress only by doing and at the same time being aware of one's actions and how they interact with events, and by simultaneously adjusting those actions in order to discover and/or achieve one's goal. It is also something that can only be learnt by doing it first, because the learning and the knowing-how comes, first of all, as a result of doing. The knowing is, in that sense, in the doing. But learning to become proficient in *professional* activity, because it involves an important moral dimension, involves more than the practice alone. It involves gaining insight into that practice by means of investigating it, reflecting upon it, theorizing about it, and challenging it with other perspectives (from formal theory or the thinking of others) and considering its moral significance and implications, in order to improve future practice.

Note: we are sharply aware that learning *professional* practice involves problems whose solution is never so clear-cut as that of Task 3.1, and that there is a danger in pressing the example too far. However, it is as yet the best vehicle we have found for unearthing a number of important issues. Before proceeding, readers should now try Task 3.1.

Unearthing meaning from the experience

If you have had some struggle with the practical task, do not seek to minimize or hide this. Your problems and your emotional (affective) reaction are an important dimension. Being willing to open up these issues and consider them openly is a vital part of working with practitioners. Maynard and Furlong highlight the point well in relation to teacher training:

> Learning to teach, as we all know but often fail to remember, is a complex, bewildering and sometimes painful task. It involves developing a practical knowledge base, changes in cognition, developing interpersonal skills and also incorporates an affective aspect (Maynard and Furlong, 1993, p. 69).

Task 3.1 Points for action

NB: The task described below is solvable. Most adults take approximately 20 minutes (children often take less). You need no resources except three friends and a place to stand in a line. Please do not write anything down as this would change the nature of the problem.

1 Find three other people to work with (children of age 9 or above or non-professional friends are quite appropriate if you cannot find colleagues). Stand in a straight line side by side.
2 Each choose a different, single syllable sound which you can make on a number of occasions. That sound is yours. It will be used to identify you. Be sure that you each choose a different one. Never let anyone else use yours.
3 Starting from one end of your line, each in turn make your sound. This will produce a pattern of sounds. Try it several times always starting from the same end of the line and always following on in the same order.
4 The people on each end of the line should now change place *with the person next to them*. (The inner two will now be on the ends) (This is called 'twiddle the ends'). When you have done this, make your own sound, still starting from the same end and following along in order as before. This will produce a new pattern of sounds.
5 Now the two (new) people in the middle should change places (those on the ends staying where they are). (This is called 'twiddle the middle'). When you have made the move, again make the new pattern of sounds, starting from the same end as always and each person still making the sound they first chose. This will produce a new pattern of sounds.
6 Continue in the following sequence: twiddle the ends and make the new pattern of sounds, keeping the sound you first chose and starting as ever from whoever is now at the original end of the line. Then twiddle the middle and make the new pattern of sound, again starting with the person at the end of the line.
7 Continue to do this, making each move in turn followed immediately by each new pattern of sound, until you come to an appropriate stopping place. (You will know when to stop.)
8 Return to your very first places.
9 *The challenge is to produce the ever-changing pattern of sounds made as if you had moved following the rules above, but continuing to stand only in your original place.*

Summary of the rules: keep to your own sound, do not write anything down, 'twiddle the ends' and make the sounds, and 'twiddle the middle' and make the sounds.
Helpful hints:
1 Be *sure* that you are following the instructions. Help each other to do so.
2 Try producing just the first two sequences of sounds without moving from your starting place. This will give you a feel for what is required.
3 Do not be afraid to keep walking it through (going back to the concrete moves).
4 You will only learn to do this by doing it. Talking will not work as a substitute for doing. Return to the text only when you have produced a performance through to the last move.

T. S. Eliot reminds us in a vivid phrase that it is possible to be involved in a series of actions, but to fail to come to grips with their significance. In 'Dry Salvages' in *Four Quartets* he describes those who: 'had the experience but missed the meaning'. Russell makes the point that without careful reconsideration, 'experience often leads to ritual knowledge rather than the desired understanding of principles' (Russell, 1993a, p. 207).

The following comments are aimed at enabling the reader to unearth some meaning from the experience of this new piece of practice, and begin to perceive some of the principles upon which it was based. Thus, unearthing the meaning comes after or at best during the action – never before it (although of course one's own basic theories exist all the time and one takes them with one into the action). This means that although one can think about (theorize about) an action before doing it, learning to practice professionally must begin with action. Often the most useful theory and theorizing for achieving action comes *during* the action as well as after it. To some extent the piece of action (practical problem) was only a vehicle for enabling us to consider: how professionals learn practice; what is involved in learning and developing practice; and how supervisors can help practitioners to profit from learning the practice of their profession. The issues raised during the period of reflection upon your new practice will include:

- the nature of learning (as a practical problem-solving activity involving people)
- what can be said about ourselves as learners (and what might be true for others)
- the nature of professional activities
- the role of the professional in practical professional problem-solving
- issues in theory and practice (the primacy of practice)
- reflection and reflective practice.

Looking back then on the practical experience, and preferably discussing it with a friend, consider first the questions in Task 3.2 and read the comments only subsequently.

Issues in learning

Most participants in this task will have discovered, perhaps with some surprise, that they have learnt to do something new, i.e. learnt new procedural knowledge (the task), and at the same time that they have learnt some new factual (propositional) knowledge, in the shape of a number of rules that were not given at the start – for example, where to stop in the sequence, and what happens to the people when they get to

---

Task 3.2 Points for considering the above task
(alone or with a colleague)

1 What do you know *now* that you did not know before? (facts/procedures?)
2 Where did that knowledge come from?
3 How did you crack this problem? (Many problems cannot be cracked of course)
4 By what processes did you learn to do it? (Did you all learn in the same way?)
   - what exactly have you learnt? (about the task, yourself, learning.)
   - what did you do?
   - what are the differences between your way of learning and the ways of others?
   - from whom did you learn to crack it? (from 'teacher'/book/from others?)
   - from whom were you *willing* to learn? (whom did you listen to?)
   - how did you feel?
   - what theories/beliefs were you working to (about yourself/others)?
   - what theories *underlay* your actions?
   - did you experience 'cognitive dissonance' (believing one thing and doing another)?
   - what are the possible differences between how you learnt and how someone watching you might learn?

---

each end of the row. This is because what they were given was a skeleton framework only, not a series of detailed moves. Most importantly, they will have discovered that they had to oscillate on a number of occasions between returning to the concrete and reworking the physical moves and then trying again to recreate the pattern of sounds at the abstract level. This is an important issue in learning something practical. In learning practical things, not only children but adults also need to go back much more frequently to the concrete than Piaget has led us all to believe. Equally important is the fact that much of the knowledge involved in cracking the problem has come from the *learner* and the interaction of one learner with another, and has not been *given* by 'teacher'. During that interaction there will have been emotional reactions also, which will have affected both the choice of whom was listened to, and how the learning proceeded (usually in fits and starts).

Further, the activity is both an individual activity and also a group one. The more the group was prepared to take risks the more quickly it will have found ways of cracking the problem. Every learner will have learnt differently. Every learner will have uncovered some tacit knowledge – some things about him or herself, about his or her views about how he or she learns and thus about how other people might learn (see Mattingly and Fleming, 1994, pp. 22–7 for a useful exposition of tacit knowledge). Every group attempting to crack the problem will have found their own group way of doing so. Anyone watching rather than doing would have had a very different experience from those participating. Anyone attempting to crack the problem by means of writing would immediately render it a different (non-practical) problem. Anyone attempting to *train* people to produce the end result would again create a very different kind of learning and a very different meaning would then emerge.

Clearly, then, the only way to learn the activity is by *doing* it. No amount of talking about it renders it any more achievable. In our culture we would often prefer to talk rather than do, because we value scientific knowledge and verbal explanation, and knowledge that is implicit and dependent on sensory experience is often considered inferior (see Mattingly and Fleming, 1994, p. 29). In fact learning to do depends upon putting action first. And 'doing' here involves concrete doing – trying out various techniques, thinking critically about them and being willing to drop them if they do not work. In short this is about improvising, reading the situation and rethinking it, and this is happening while participants are on their feet, moving and making sounds all at the same time. As we shall see later, this is what Schön refers to as 'thinking-in-action' and 'knowing-in-action' (see Schön, 1987, chapter 2).

It is also important to note, however, that in considering this activity, some people will argue that a detailed analysis of what has happened during this learning is only achievable up to a point. For them there is to some extent a mystery in how the final performance has been achieved. They consider that it is not possible to recreate totally all the fleeting thoughts and actions in the order that they happened, or to know exactly how certain ideas suddenly emerged. Others, however, believe that you can atomize the events down to the last single action, plot the moves and then teach them to others. These two extreme views arise from the two polar approaches to professional practice described in Chapter 2. The considerable importance of this for trying to understand how practitioners learn to practice will be considered in the next section of this chapter.

Let us now turn to issues about supervision which also lie embedded in the experience. Consider first the questions in Task 3.3 which focus upon our role as 'teachers' in setting up this problem and in helping learners to unearth the meaning from it.

Task 3.3 Points for consideration
(alone or with a colleague)

1 What have been the various roles of the 'teacher' in this practical problem-solving activity?
2 What might they involve in real practice as opposed to how we have to work because this is a book?
3 What were our intentions in setting up this problem for you?
4 What sorts of supervision strategies are involved in using a problem-solving situation?
5 Where does 'authority' reside in the activity?
6 Was it in the same place throughout? (What did you take on trust? What did you challenge?)

Issues in supervision

When we offer this activity as part of clinical supervision workshops, we start by using four volunteers to demonstrate the task. This is because in a workshop everything is done orally and demonstrations help to make the task clear, which is more important when participants have no instructions to refer back to as the reader has here. These demonstrations do *not*, however, offer a model to be followed. They merely offer a picture of the rules. In fact we stop the demonstration before the entire sequence has been revealed. It is an interesting issue to consider exactly what role demonstration plays in supervision. This will be taken up in the next new section below.

During and after the demonstrations we work hard to get participants to trust us and to be willing to have a go at the task. This is because they cannot yet know about the use of this task as a vehicle to reach issues that lie deeper (and so the task might seem trivial), and because we must set an atmosphere in which it is safe to take risks, to get it wrong, to try again, to profit from mistakes and to see them as growing points. We also have to ensure that everyone has equal rights to their opinions and to their own ways of doing things, in order that everyone will feel safe to learn. We cannot do some of these things so easily via the printed word, but you might like to consider how we have tried to do some of it.

It is important to notice the minimal role of instructions in the activity. We said above that what we offered was a mere skeleton of rules. Certainly we offered you nine points and four hints. But we also believed that you would find certain things out for yourselves and in doing so would own them more fully than you would if we had told you them. The supervisor here has to trust the participants to draw upon a range of pre-existing knowledge and to be able to uncover it in order to crack the problem. Such an approach is important too in dealing with practitioners who come with a wealth of experience to the process of continued development as a practitioner.

This means that the supervisor who uses practical problem-solving gives up the authority role in order to become an enabler, to set the scene in a supportive way and to encourage the learners to draw upon their own resources. The locus of authority then resides not in the supervisor, who, in the workshop version of this task, stands at the back rather than the front during the demonstration, who focuses the class on the demonstrating quartet, who sends fours off to practise privately, and who leads the reflections afterwards by means of questions rather than statements. The locus of authority is, rather, with the learners. During practice the group discovers that authority resides in different learners at different points in the process. The negotiation of this between learners is of considerable interest in terms of group dynamics, since quite often an individual discovers with some horror that they have attempted to take the group over or to impose on someone else a learning style that is inappropriate for them. Quite often, too, a group in difficulties only cracks it when one individual having trouble eventually rejects the dominance of another who has sought to impose one way of learning on everyone, and strikes out for his or her own way of doing it.

All this raises some very interesting issues about theory and practice. The following section seeks to explore this.

Theory and practice

The role of theory in practical affairs is in fact central, as was indicated at the beginning of this chapter and as Wilfred Carr and Eraut also point out (see below). For our purposes (for the moment) there are two main kinds of theory. Formal theory is formulated and argued for publicly, is commonly known and generally (if temporarily) accepted as current thinking (which is sometimes mistaken for proven fact). Personal theory is a mixture of beliefs and assumptions, values and private theories, perhaps influenced by formal theory, and cashing out into everyday practice. Carr, by reference to teaching, draws our attention to the elements of formal theory which can influence practice, but notes how in practice it is transmuted by personal theory:

> what is distinctive of an educational practice is that it is guided, not just by some general practical theory, but also by the exigencies of the practical situation in which this theory is to be applied. Thus, the guidance given by theory always has to be moderated by the guidance given by *phronesis* – wise and prudent judgement about if, and to what extent, this 'theory' ought to be invoked and enacted in a concrete case (W. Carr, 1987, pp. 172–3).

Eraut focuses on personal theory. He makes the points that when people start using a theory they stop calling it a theory, and that people become alienated by 'theory' as a result of being constantly subjected to other people's rather than being encouraged to develop (or to recognize) their own. He adds:

> Yet people use theory all the time; and it is their personal theories which determine how they interpret the world and their encounters with people and situations within it (Eraut, 1989, p. 184).

Within personal theory, Argyris and Schön make a useful distinction between espoused theories (the theories of action to which we give allegiance when asked to say what we believe) and theories-in-use (the theories that actively govern our actions) (see Argyris and Schön, 1974, pp. 6–7). This often leads to the difference between knowing what one should do and doing something else. How espoused theories become theories-in-use is an interesting question.

Task 3.4 Points for consideration
(alone or with a colleague)

1 What espoused theories did you bring to this practice (about yourself; learning, problem-solving)?
2 What 'theories-in-use' lay under your actions? Did both sets of theories match?
3 How will the experience influence your future practice, your views about theory, and your own theories?

Many participants in the above problem-solving exercise realize, on looking back at it, that they had begun the task with a number of theories about, for example, how to solve such problems, how to tackle this particular one, how they can best learn, what the task is really about. In some cases participants will have begun with some theories about how a tutor involved in post-registration education or in-service provision should operate during a workshop or an author should behave in a book (and therefore how a practising professional should be expected to learn), and have found these to be in contrast to the practice associated with this task. The reader may even have felt surprise as we flouted some of the conventions of writing a book by sending the audience away from the text to carry out some practice. As Schön points out, surprise is a useful signal to attend to in trying to explore and improve practice. It often draws attention to the unexpected, and this in turn often marks the existence of a conflict between belief and action (a challenge to practice by theory, or vice versa) (see Schön, 1987, pp. 26–8).

During the trial and error of the activity, no doubt assorted theories conflicted both internally within individuals and externally between group members, and probably theory was modified by practice and vice versa. While all of these theories-in-action are held fluidly, while theory is remembered to be unproven ideas and while participants are willing to adjust their ideas and their practices according to the needs of the specific piece of practice, both theory and practice can refine each other. Eraut, who looks at the problems of analysing teaching, refers to the importance of 'flexibility, adaptability, situational understanding and ability to learn from experience'. He also makes the point (quoting Nisbitt and Ross, 1980) that: 'there is a considerable body of psychological evidence to show that personal theories have a significant effect on how people think, act and perform' (see Eraut, 1989, p. 184). This is all true for both practitioners and their supervisors.

Recognizing the theories upon which one is working provides one with the power to 'bring the largely intuitive aspects of . . . practice under some kind of critical control'. He adds, significantly:

> Once one becomes more aware of the nature and effect of one's own theories, then it is possible to also consider those of others, whether they be immediate colleagues or authors of books. Similarly, by recognising the contexts in which one has developed one's theories, one is better able to judge when new theories are needed to cope with new kinds of contexts (Eraut, 1989, p. 184).

Eraut also highlights the role of theory in strategic thinking, which requires an understanding of the context, a set of priorities, awareness of alternatives and an ability to predict the consequences of various courses of action over the longer term. Participants in the set task may see, on looking back over it, that they did indeed draw upon these and as a result did initiate or abort particular attempts at action. But it is in fact very difficult to 'see' or to trace such happening by observation unless it enters the discussion between group members and that discussion is recorded.

All of this strongly challenges the notion of the supervisor simply telling a practitioner how to operate. It could also be argued that reflection is a tool of investigation. Such issues are taken up in Chapter 5. It is first necessary to clarify the ideas involved and to relate them to the task given above.

Reflective practice

All the activities and discussions in the three sub-sections above have been versions of or approaches to reflection on practice. Without such

---

Task 3.5 Points for consideration
(alone or with a colleague)

1 List briefly the things you have learnt as a result of the reflections prompted above.
2 How have these reflections affected your understanding of the experience of the task?
3 What do you understand by reflection on practice, and what processes are involved in it?
4 How might what you have learnt through practice today relate to your later professional practice?

---

processes, the meaning and significance of the task would probably have lain dormant in the minds of readers and thus never impacted upon future practice. For this reason reflection is, for those who subscribe to the professional artistry view, a central tool in learning through practice. For those whose supervision is guided by a technical–rational approach, of course, telling and training are what matter. Our argument, however, is that that approach may make for short-term efficiency, but that it deprives practitioners of individuality and of the means of developing and improving their practice in the longer term.

Reflection itself is about reconsidering – even 're-seeing' – practice. It is located within the tradition of experiential learning (see Kolb, 1984; Osterman and Kottkamp, 1993, p. 20), and can happen both during and after the action. (There can be consideration of action beforehand which also involves some imagined viewing of what is intended, or some reconsideration of previous practice.)

Reflection may involve a number of processes. There is no simple set pattern for this – that is one of its strengths (though it often involves the four elements of Kolb's experiential learning theory: concrete experience; observation and analysis (or interpretation); abstract reconceptualization; and active experimentation) (see Kolb, 1984; Osterman and Kottkamp, 1993, p. 20). What can be said, however, is that any systematic approach to reflection can be used to investigate and theorize about practice. The process of reflection enables critical consideration of practice and its moral dimensions. This does presuppose a seeking rather than a knowing attitude to practice and to one's responsibilities within practice, and thus it requires the practitioner to be open to criticism and to the possible need to change. What it does not do is to provide a clear set of detailed instructions for carrying out new practice. In that it is tentative and enquiring rather than assertive about knowledge, reflection is very much against the prevailing climate of our (rather unintelligent) times, where certainty of intention and achievement and simplicity of skills and procedures seem to be expected in every occupation irrespective of the nature of that occupation.

Reflective practice, then, is about using reflection to enlighten, develop and improve professional action. It is 'an empowering and motivational process' and enables individuals to be more effective and assume greater responsibility for their own practices (Osterman and Kottkamp, 1993, p. 185), and it takes both practice and theory seriously (see Golby, 1993a, p. 41).

Systematic reflection, of course, does not come naturally. As Mickan notes, there needs to be an explicit commitment for students to reflect (Mickan, 1995, p. 243). However, the ability to reflect, to share those reflections and, for supervisors, to lead others to reflect, is crucially dependent not only on knowing about reflection, but also on having a language – or being confident enough to create or invent a language – in which to reflect. Mattingly and Fleming in their major research on occupational therapy in America discovered this too. They say:

> We did not know when we began this research study that one thing we had to offer therapists was a foreign language that they could use to examine their own practice, seeing familiar things in a new way.

They also make the point that an observer (or supervisor) can aid this process of seeing anew.

> The external viewer forces people to talk in a different language. Thus they [the observed therapists] have to think about [their practice] differently and reformulate their notions to explain them in a language the observer can understand.

They add:

> The development of a common language, which helped [therapists] to recognize and then to articulate the large body of tacit knowledge they had in common, was seen as an extraordinary asset, not only to their practice per se, but to their recognition as professionals in their work settings (Mattingly and Fleming, 1994, pp. 14–15).

Schön has provided us with some important (if controversial and incomplete) notions and some useful language in which to distinguish two different kinds of reflection. These he calls reflection-in-action and reflection-on-action.

He relates the first of these to what he calls *knowing-in-action*. By this he means the kinds of knowledge we show in our intelligent action. He cites public, observable actions like riding a bicycle and private actions like analysing a balance sheet. In both cases he maintains, the knowing is in the action. And we show the existence of such knowing through our spontaneous, skilful carrying out of the performance. The processes involved in such knowing-in-action, however, are often unable to be made verbally explicit but can sometimes be observed or reflected on afterwards in order to describe the tacit knowing embedded in them. For example we can uncover the sequences of our procedures and processes and the rules we follow, as well as our values, beliefs and personal theories, all of which are given away by overt clues. Schön argues that:

> whatever language we employ, however, our descriptions of knowing-in-action are always *constructions*. They are always attempts to put into explicit, symbolic form a kind of intelligence that begins by being tacit and spontaneous. Our descriptions are conjectures that need to be tested against observations of their originals – which, in at least one respect, they are bound to distort. For knowing-in-action is dynamic, and 'facts', 'procedures', 'rules', and 'theories' are static (Schön, 1987, p. 25).

Schön goes on to explain how in response to the jolt of the unexpected during a piece of action, we may reflect upon the incident by looking back upon it, or we may pause in the midst of action (but now outside it) to think what we should do next (Schön, 1987, pp. 27–31). These are both examples of *reflection-on-action*, in which we relate (to a piece of practice we have recently executed), some ordered, deliberate and systematic questions about practice, which arise specifically from that practice. There is no set version of this and reflection can utilize a range of different processes, chosen for their appropriateness to the specific piece of practice. Without much conscious experience of this process, however, practitioners are inclined to reflect in a totally haphazard way, seizing on any aspect of the practice that first comes to mind. Readers may have done this in moments when they stopped their actions in the given task and discussed what to do next. For this reason a systematic approach to reflection is needed. But it must be one which allows the user to be responsive to the specific and unique characteristics of the activity under consideration. A flexible framework rather than a set of routines is therefore needed. One such is offered and considered in detail in Chapter 6.

Of *reflection-in-action*, on the other hand, Schön says:

> When we have learned how to do something, we can execute smooth sequences of activity, recognition, decision, and adjustment without having, as we say, to 'think about it'.

(Readers may not have reached that stage with the task set above, but if they practised it for long enough it would happen.) Schön goes on:

> Our spontaneous knowing-in-action usually gets us through the day. On occasion, however, it doesn't. A familiar routine produces an unexpected result; an error stubbornly resists correction. . . . All such experiences . . . contain an element of *surprise* (Schön, 1987, p. 26).

Then, we may reflect in the middle of the action (while we can still make a difference to the action we are involved in and *without interrupting it*. This is reflection-in-action. In this case, and simultaneously with continuing the action, we perceive a puzzle, and invent and implement solutions, using on-the-spot experimentation and trial and error which is not random, and which involves critical questioning of the assumptions and structure of knowing-in-action. This process includes restructuring both our strategies and also our very thinking about the action and our understanding of it. Schön talks here of 'ways of reframing problems'. Readers will probably have experienced such processes during the set task. Reflection-in-action, then, has immediate significance for action, and is even coincidental with it. Schön maintains that a skilled performer can adjust his responses to variations which occur moment-by-moment, and integrate reflection-in-action into a smooth performance of an ongoing task.

Russell and Munby, who have worked on Schön's ideas and their use in teacher training for many years, characterize reflection-in-action as 'a process with non-logical features that is prompted by experience and over which we have limited control' (Russell and Munby, 1991, p. 164). For them 'the essence of reflection-in-action is 're-framing' (Schön's term), which means the 'hearing' or 'seeing differently', in which observation is interpretative rather than analytical. Reframing, they say, 'mediates between theory and practice, revealing new meanings in theory and new strategies for practice' (Russell and Munby, 1991, p. 166). They add, however, that a new frame does not mean an end to puzzles and problems, but that the 'scrutiny of one's own practice continues . . . [and] moves on to more elaborated views of practice' (p. 173). Their research so far has led them to view the reframing of puzzling experiences, particularly those about the inconsistency of theory and practice, as very significant in developing teachers' professional knowledge and action. They also note that revised theories-in-action are accompanied by changes in the teachers' descriptive language.

Seeking consistency between theory and practice and better theories to guide practice appears to be an important element in productive reframing (Russell and Munby, 1991, p. 184).

Schön himself translates all of this into a professional context, discussing professional practice as opposed to a practical problem like making a gate (Schön, 1987, chapter 2). We shall pick up his fourth notion – that of *knowing-in-practice* (where practice refers to professional practice as a whole) in the section below.

Task 3.6 Points for consideration
(alone or with a colleague)

So far we have discussed the practical task given at the start of this chapter under the headings: learning; supervising; theory and practice; and reflecting on practice.

1 Review in your mind what you have learnt about each of these four.
2 List briefly the implications of the given task and these discussions of it for *clinical supervision.*
3 You may like to compare your list with that which comes towards the end of the next section.

Practice in a professional setting

Learning professional practice

So far we have considered a practical problem-solving task which can be solved. This task, though a practical one, is not strictly a professional one, though it is closely related to the nature of professional practice in its requirement for collaborative learning and in that it can only be learnt by doing. Some of the main differences, however, between it and a professional activity aimed at learning to practise are:

1 that the task was an individual 'one-off' activity
2 that the set task was susceptible to solution
3 that, although the means by which people learn to do it are variable, the solution (final performance) has the same surface features for everyone, everywhere
4 that there is nothing contestable about the solution, which receives universal agreement
5 that there were no moral complexities about the solution.

By contrast, solutions to individual activities in professional practice are best understood from within that tradition; are at best temporary (can never be fully solved); are situation specific; are essentially contestable (because value-related); and have a moral dimension. Indeed, professional practice is an open capacity, cannot be mastered and goes on being refined for ever. (Arguably there is a major onus on supervisors to demonstrate this and to reveal its implications in their own practice.)

As Michael Golby points out, in the term 'professional practice' the word 'practice' refers not to an individual activity but, to a 'whole tradition in which particular activities are related together as part of a social project or mission' (Golby, 1993a, p. 4). For education, the social project is the promotion of knowledge, just as for the legal profession it is justice and for the medical profession it is health. He also makes the point that professional practice is not value-free (see also Chapter 1).Values, as he points out, though they underlie the daily activities of practitioners, are not delivered as end products. 'Discussion of values and principles is therefore best conducted in the context of specific professional activities'. He goes on to make the point that professional practice:

> is not merely habitual skilled behaviour but a stream of highly miscellaneous activities unified as serving a social good. Practice has a history which can be seen as the collective pursuit of human good; as an historic phenomenon, practices have their own language and style. Though there are of necessity routine and unreflecting parts of daily professional life, loss of sight of fundamental values which have evolved historically in the activities of practice is at once a loss of professionalism (Golby, 1993a, p. 5).

He also offers us the important understanding that just as the unique speaking of an individual relies upon the pre-existence of our own language (which comes to us as received tradition of expression, carrying cultural traditions), so (for example) 'educational practice has its own history and culture in which individual practitioners partici-pate' and which they express in their own way. Thus, learning to become a professional is 'a matter of coming ever more fully into membership of a tradition of practice' and, 'at its maturity it is a matter of taking part in more fully shaping practice for the future'. This involves understanding the inherited traditions of a profession (and/or of the preparation to enter that profession), and considering critically and practically their present relevance (see Golby, 1993a, p. 8).

We therefore need to consider what can now be said about the processes of learning professional practice and exactly what we can

draw from our discussions of the set task to enlighten our understanding of learning professional practice and of enabling others to
learn and develop it.

The philosophical bases of learning professional practice

The nature of professional practice, then, is that it is social, moral and
complex, and is embedded in traditions of practice. It cannot be
mastered. We can already say that learning professional practice is
achieved by learning through experience. What can we say then about
this idea and its history?

The notion of learning through experience goes back to the Greeks,
where it was shaped by Aristotle's notions of 'praxis' and practical
reasoning, and comes to us more immediately via Dewey, Van Manen,
Schwab, Stenhouse and Schön. These, then, are the thinkers who have
shaped the traditions which supervisors are now taking on. Evidence of
the influence of their ideas can be found, for example, in the work of
Mattingly and Fleming on clinical reasoning. They maintain that: 'clinical reasoning in occupational therapy is quite close to Aristotle's ancient
concept of practical reasoning' (Mattingly and Fleming, 1994, p. 10); and
that: 'clinical reasoning for occupational therapists was not simply scientific reasoning, matching condition to therapy ... it went beyond that to
a complex practical reasoning aimed at determining 'the good' for each
particular 'patient' (Mattingly and Fleming, 1994, p. 13). The influence
of their work is fast spreading across health care professions.

Wilfred Carr, by reference to Aristotle, points out that the Greek
word *praxis* means roughly the same as our term 'practice', though the
classical context in which it existed gave it a different dimension. Thus
praxis is a way of distinguishing 'doing something' from *poesis*, 'making
something'. The end of *poesis* is an object which is known prior to the
action, and the processes involved in this production are guided by a
form of knowledge which Aristotle calls *techne* – which we would now
call technical knowledge. *Poesis* is a species of rule-following action.
Carr reminds us that for Aristotle the activities of shipbuilder,
craftsmen and artisans were paradigm cases of *poesis* guided by *techne*.
Praxis is also directed to the achievement of an end, not a concrete end
but the end of 'some morally worthwhile good'. Such good cannot be
made. It can only be done. Practice is thus a form of 'doing (moral)
action', whose end can only be realized through action, and can only
exist in action. These ends are not immutable and fixed. They cannot be
specified in advance of the action. They are what they are at the time
and can only be understood in terms of the tradition in which the good
intrinsic to practice is enshrined. He says that a practice:

is always the achievement of a tradition, and it is only by submitting to its authority that practitioners can begin to acquire the practical knowledge and standards of excellence by means of which their own practical competence can be judged. But the authoritative nature of a tradition does not make it immune to criticism. The practical knowledge made available through tradition is not simply reproduced; it is also constantly re-interpreted and revized through dialogue and discussion about how to pursue the practical goods which constitute the tradition (W. Carr, 1987, pp. 169–70).

Thus, he argues, by a process of a critical reconstruction the tradition evolves and changes.

Dewey is the modern philosopher whose ideas about learning through experience have provided the foundations for practical-based education in the twentieth century. It is in highlighting the fact that professional practice is the province of a community of practitioners who share the traditions of a calling, that part of Dewey's contribution to our thinking is made. He also offers us perspectives on the knowledge needed and the processes involved in learning through practice. He it was who first discussed reflective practice, and distinguished between routine (unthinking) actions and reflective actions which show awareness of the principles and grounds of our practices, and who pointed out that systematic enquiry into practice is necessary to bring this fully to consciousness, in order that we have a secure understanding of the grounds of our actions (see Dewey, 1933).

Van Manen's work is important in offering an early model of reflection. His view of reflection is hierarchical. He suggests three levels of reflection, the first being concerned with technical/practical details, the second with assumptions that underlie action and underpin the value of competing educational goals, and the third with moral and ethical issues (see Van Manen (1990) in which he reiterates his original contribution). He is critical of action research that simply slips from reflection-on-action straight to problem-solving, and emphasizes the second and third levels of reflection as essential.

Schwab has developed our ideas in respect of deliberation, which is a kind of public and social form of reflection aimed particularly at decision-making about curriculum design and evaluation (see Schwab, 1969).

Stenhouse developed the important notion of the teacher as researcher (Stenhouse, 1975), now developed further into the enquiring teacher by the work of, for example, Elliott, Hopkins, Nias, and Rudduck. He argued for the 'emancipation' of practitioners by encouraging them to adopt the perspective of researchers. The process of being a practitioner-researcher would, he believed, strengthen professionals' judgement and lead to the self-directed improvement of practice. Accordingly, his many and powerful writings about research (focusing, for example, on what counts as research, the role of research in professional practice, and the case-study tradition), published between the late 1970s and, posthumously, the mid-1980s, have provided an important basis for helping reflective practitioners to investigate their practice (see Rudduck and Hopkins, 1985, p. 3). For him the means to professional development for practitioners was a research process in which they systematically reflected on their practice and used the results to improve such practice. (See the notion of taking an investigative stance towards teaching in Chapter 4.) Stenhouse also subscribed to the notion of the practitioner as artist in which 'ideas and action are fused' in the practice of one's own performance. Comparing the art of practice with artistry generally he wrote of the development of art as 'a dialectic of ideas and practice not to be separated from change'. He added of art:

> Exploration and interpretation lead to revision and adjustment of idea and of practice . . . look at the sketch book of a good artist, a play in rehearsal, a jazz quartet working together. That, I am arguing, is what good teaching [professional practice] is like. . . .
>   Note, however, that the process of developing the art of the artist is always associated with change in ideas and practice. . . . There is no mastery, always aspiration. And the aspiration is about ideas – content, as well as about performance – execution of ideas (Stenhouse in Rudduck and Hopkins, 1985, p. 97).

Schön extends these ideas about artistry, considering matters like improvisation and its role, but most importantly he has analysed technical rationality and found it wanting on three counts:

1 it ignores the extent to which professional knowledge is and must be exercised in the institutional settings particular to the profession
2 it is indifferent to the way professionals actually work
3 it underrates the messy complexity of practice (see Schön, 1983, 1987).

Most importantly, though, and because he rejects the technical–rational approach, Schön has contributed to our development of an epistemology of practice, and to our developing language of reflection.

> If the model of Technical Rationality . . . fails to account for practical competence in divergent situations, so much the worse for the model. Let us search instead for an epistemology of practice implicit in artistic, intuitive processes which some practitioners do bring to situ-

ations of uncertainty, instability, uniqueness and value conflict (Schön, 1983, p. 49).

We have already looked at some of Schön's central concepts in his theory of knowledge of practice and consider others below. Before moving to these, however, we should note that Schön's work is a beginning, not an end. He has begun a process which needs much more work before we have a full sense of how knowing-in-practice operates, and even then we shall not be able to analyse it absolutely nor shall we master it. What Schön offers, then, is ideas on which practitioners need to work. However, there are a number of critics of his work – many of whom view professional practice in a more technical–rational way. For example, Gilroy is unhappy about the varying uses of the term 'reflection' and what he sees as the unhelpfulness of uncertainty. He (rightly in our view) sees the possibilities of infinite regression in an undisciplined version of reflection which omits discussion of wider issues, including moral aspects, and which ignores the contribution to thinking of the views and ideas of others (see Gilroy, 1993). Gilroy prefers, for example, the work of Stones and sees teaching as a game in which the rules should be defined. (This raises interesting questions not only about what such rules consist of and how to gain consensus for all but the most general, but also about whether artistry involves playing creatively within rules or finding creative expression that goes beyond them. It is thus not clear how far this analogy can be taken.) Eraut (1995), in an article entitled 'Schön shock: a case for reframing reflection in action?', concludes that 'most of Schön's examples fail to provide evidence of reflection-in-action', but rather relate to reflection-on-action, and offers three recommendations for reframing Schön's account (Eraut, 1995, p. 9). Van Manen raises questions about the meaning and place of practical reflection in teaching (Van Manen, 1995). Hartley (1993) also sees reflective practice as undesirable in that it often operates only at a descriptive level. However, like the reservations of Gilroy, Eraut and Van Manen, these are not about the work of Schön, but about the problems that occur when it is misused.

Task 3.7 Points for consideration (alone or with a colleague)

1 Review in your mind what you have learnt from the brief history of ideas offered in this sub-section.
2 How do they relate to those offered in Chapter 2?

Some key concepts in learning professional practice

Learning professional practice, then, though complex and never entirely able to be analysed, clearly involves learning through experience. A number of concepts associated with this have been usefully elucidated by Schön (1983, 1987), and some of them have been explored further by Russell (see Russell, 1993a).

Schön has highlighted knowing-in-action; reflection-in-action; and reflection-on-action; and he has called attention to the importance of puzzles and surprises and to the notion of reframing. In learning practice Schön's idea of a *sheltered practicum* is also useful. (This is an experience of practice where the student has a taste of real practice but does not bear the full responsibility for every aspect of the work.) Schön describes the main features of a practicum as: 'learning by doing, coaching rather than teaching, and a dialogue of reciprocal reflection-in-action between coach and student' (see Schön, 1987, p. 303; see below, p. 84, for his ideas on coaching).

Russell explores the processes of learning through experience as they are related to learning to teach. He makes the point that because teacher training has lacked detail about how student teachers can learn through experience, practices developed during teaching practice 'easily become rituals without supporting principles, and theory, often seen as elaborate common sense, is comprehended but not related to practices' (Russell, 1993a, p. 209). In nursing, Walsh and Ford (1989) give similar examples of the problems of rituals informing nursing practice, while Mattingly and Fleming offer important investigations of what they call clinical reasoning.

Russell traces the problem to the fact that direct experience can lead to ritual knowledge without principled understanding, because the learner's understanding of practice remains 'at the level of specific experiences and practical procedures'. Russell highlights the usefulness for Initial Teacher Education (ITE) of notions of *ritual knowledge* (routinized know-how); and *principled knowledge* ('essentially explanatory, oriented towards understanding of how procedures and processes work, of why certain conclusions are necessary or valid rather than being arbitrary things to say because they seem to please the teacher') (see Russell, 1993a, p. 210). Russell makes the point that: 'changing one's patterns, particularly in the light of theory or research, requires knowledge of the principles implicit in the present practices, and here ritual knowledge is inadequate'. He goes on to argue that at present most teachers' practical knowledge remains ritualized, and that there are no traditions of using the observation and analysis of working teachers to enable them to move from ritual to principles. He points out that normally observation of a professional teacher is used only when they are already failing, and concludes:

> Observation of teachers by those with more experience and authority competes directly with the potential of experience to modify teachers' frames for conducting and interpreting their work. So long as teachers associate observation with the threat of potentially arbitrary criticism, the profession denies itself opportunity to discover the value of recording teaching events for subsequent review and detailed analysis, leading to understanding of the principles implicit in present practices (Russell, 1993a, p. 214).

We thus have a range of useful concepts related to learning professional practice. To these might be added the following crucial distinctions:

- learning professional practice (which means learning to operate within a tradition)
- learning from practice (which means learning by watching and perhaps copying)
- learning by practice (which means learning by endless repeating of actions)
- learning through practice (which means learning about principled actions via the learning of one specific activity).

This last version is about establishing the foundation of principled procedures, and is important because learning to bring practice under control and improve it is aided by exhuming and examining the principles underlying our actions (see Fish, 1989, chapter 4).

All of this has a number of things to tell us about how to learn professional practice and how to help practitioners develop their practice. It also offers us critical perspectives on present models of learning professional practice.

Some models of learning professional practice

There are many models proposed that purport to exemplify how professional practice might be acquired and improved. They all have the universal drawback of models in that they reduce and simplify the complexity of practice. But some offer us useful ideas – even if they are ideas that we reject – because they help us to clarify our thinking. The following outlines some of the better known ideas which are currently influencing thinking about professional education (Task 3.8).

Some models were originally devised to structure learning in a range of professions, including nursing. These are all based upon technical–

Task 3.8 Points for consideration
(alone or with a colleague)

It is instructive to ask of each model as you read, what are its underlying views about:

• the character of supervision
• practitioners as learners
• the capabilities of reflective practitioners
• how practitioners and supervisors will relate together.

---

rational notions of incremental approaches to learning practice. They assume that learners can only operate at a simple (noviciate) level in all early practice and become more dependable experts the more practice they have. Such models include that of Benner (1984), who suggests that student nurses climb gradually through a range of competencies from novice to expert, and whose work was based upon the skill acquisition model of Dreyfus and Dreyfus (1986). This influential model offers a five stage progression from novice to expert which was developed in the context of the training of aircraft pilots. Both Dreyfus and Dreyfus and Benner posit that capturing the descriptions of expert practice is important, and is possible, though difficult, because the expert 'operates from a deep understanding of the total situation' (Benner, 1984, p. 32). Though apparently less than fully technical–rational, these models run contrary to the notion of professional artistry which sees students as bringing knowledge with them, finding it in action and as being able to consider some moral dimensions of practice and deal with incidents in practice with a wisdom that is not necessarily related to length of practice. Indeed, any model is bound of its own nature to be technical–rational.

Another version, however, is found in the literature on nursing, where Bulman provides exemplars of students' reflections on their practice which in part do illustrate professional artistry but do not fully show students dealing with incidents in practice by using wisdom unrelated to their time in practice (Bulman, 1994). But in some ways the best means of characterizing professional artistry is in the 'three dimensional and human model' presented in Task 3.1 above.

We are now in a position to summarize what we might say so far about the processes through which professional practice is learnt and developed, and to distinguish the issues central to that learning.

Issues and processes useful in learning professional practice

It is, of course, only possible to say some tentative things about learning professional practice at this stage. But even these probably represent progress in our understanding compared to what it was at the start of the book (Task 3.9).

Task 3.9 Points for consideration
(alone or with a colleague)

Readers are invited:
- to consider critically the following list of points
- to compare these with their own, made in response to the task on page 51
- to reconsider the views that underlay their early responses to the exercises in Chapter 1, pp. 18 and 32.

The following summarizes some points useful in understanding how we learn professional practice:

- action comes first
- action has theories embedded in it because theory and practice are part of each other
- theory comes in a variety of forms, including personal theory and formal theory
- personal theory includes espoused theory and theories-in-use
- learners *come* with knowledge, which needs to be explored and built on
- learners often need the minimum enabling framework to start with
- there is a need to return frequently to the concrete and to oscillate between this and principles relevant to the practice (to engage in a 'dialectic of ideas and practice', in Stenhouse's terms)
- it is quite possible to move bodily, make sounds and think *at the same time*
- such 'thoughtful action' (which Schön calls knowing-in-action) often involves improvising and thinking on one's feet
- insight into action can then be gained by reflecting on, theorizing about and investigating practice
- gaining insight means unearthing the meaning, and thus the significant values and the principles, that lie beneath the actions
- to this extent any one piece of action is a vehicle for learning principles
- gaining insight into one's own actions is more important than being told by someone else what to do and how
- practical learning proceeds in fits and starts
- there is a strong affective element
- every learner will learn differently

- risk-taking is a key to successful practical problem-solving and to the more temporary problem-solving of professional practice
- talking, reading or writing about the task is no substitute for the experience of doing it (though it can aid reflection-on-action afterwards)
- being trained to do something practical is a quite different process with very different and less transferable outcomes
- the role of demonstration in learning practice need not be the same as apprenticeship. Demonstration can be used to set the problem, not show how to solve it
- it is important to set an atmosphere where risks can be taken, mistakes made, everyone has equal say
- practice needs to be observed, captured and used to work towards its informing principles
- reflection on practice may not lead to immediate visible improvement, but rather to longer-term quality in practice and professionalism.

The final question then is: what does this tell us about the skills, processes and issues necessary for a supervisor to facilitate practitioners' learning through practice?

Issues and processes useful in supervising a professional practitioner

Basically a supervisor is someone who enables a practitioner to learn and develop through practice. So far then, we can say the following kinds of things about the skills and knowledge a supervisor needs for this enterprise:

- the locus of knowledge for succeeding in the situation is in the practitioner not in the supervisor
- in order to enable the practitioner to learn and develop through practice, the supervisor often has to give up authority, and know how to hand it over to the practitioner
- the supervisor needs to know how to reflect on practice, know how to investigate practice, know the role of puzzles in learning, and how theory and practice refine each other
- the supervisor needs to be willing to demonstrate that his or her own practice is developed and refined by these very approaches
- the supervisor needs to be a seeker rather than a knower about professional practice, and to be comfortable enough with uncertainty to be able to share it
- the supervisor needs to be open to criticism and change
- the supervisor needs to help the practitioner to learn from the successes and failures of their own practice
- the supervisor needs to be able to talk with practitioners about

competence but also be able to focus them on the competencies required by the profession, and further, ought to be able to enable them to develop their own agendas in respect of competence and competencies

- the supervisor needs to help practitioners to learn not only from their strengths but also from their problems
- on each occasion where the supervisor works with a practitioner, although there may be a need to focus on specific predetermined aspects of practice, supervisors also ought to be prepared to respond to other major issues as they arise
- the supervisor needs to enable practitioners to recognize successful strategies but also to encourage them to learn others (and thus to widen their repertoire)
- the supervisor needs to help practitioners to test the adequacy of their practices and to make explicit their criteria for this
- the supervisor needs to enable practitioners to learn the skills, understandings and attitudes necessary in order to continue their own professional development (adapted from McIntyre and Haggar, 1993, pp. 91–3).

The literature of mentoring in Initial Teacher Education is full of articles proposing various models of supervision (Fish, 1989; Dunne and Dunne, 1993; Dunne and Harvard, 1993; McIntyre and Haggar, 1993; Maynard and Furlong, 1993), but many are formulations of fairly obvious approaches to supervision.

However, it is Schön who offers one of the most useful perspectives on supervisor behaviour in his models of coaching. He describes the coach's skill as operating in one of three models, which he emphasizes are ideal types and may in reality occur in one session. These models are: 'joint experimentation'; 'follow me'; and 'hall of mirrors'. Here the dialogue of coach and student calls for different sorts of improvisation, presents different orders of difficulty and lends itself to different contexts.

Joint experimentation is useful when the student already knows what he or she wants to produce. Here the coach first helps the student to formulate the qualities he or she wants to achieve and then by demonstration or description explores different ways of producing them. The skills here involve leading the student to search for ways of operating. The student has to be willing to have a go. The coach 'works at creating and sustaining a process of collaborative enquiry', and must resist the temptation to tell the student how to do it – though he can perhaps generate some solutions and enable the student to choose (Schön, 1987, p. 296).

When the coach wants to offer a new way of seeing and doing things, the *follow me* approach is apparently more useful. Here the coach improvises 'a whole designlike performance', and offers examples of reflection-in-action. The coach is able to take a holistic view of the action, to break it up into various aspects and to reassemble it. He demonstrates and then responds to the student's attempts to imitate him. There is danger of confusion and ambiguity, so the coach uses all kinds of language and analogies and the student tries to follow him, attempting to construct his or her own meanings (see Schön, 1987, p. 296). In its pure form, this model is more useful for working with health practitioners than for coaching student teachers, but in its indication of ways of helping practitioners to reflect, it is generally important, and its spirit is caught by the framework for reflection offered in Chapter 6.

In *hall of mirrors* 'student and coach continually shift perspective' (see Schön, 1987, p. 297). They shift from re-enacting the student's practice to dialogue about it, to redesigning it. Here there is 'a premium on the coach's ability to surface his own confusions'. This model can only be created, Schön says, when there are close parallels between the practicum and real practice – when the coaching resembles the interpersonal practice to be learned. This is therefore a useful approach for clinical supervision.

Schön also makes the important point that when coach and student do their jobs well they act as 'on-line researchers, each enquiring more or less consciously into his own and the other's changing understandings'. But it is clear that there can be no mastery of this. 'The behavioural world of the practicum is complex, variable and resistant to control' (see Schön, 1987, p. 298). The best that can be achieved is a willing cooperation in trying to grasp one's own and others' understandings. This understanding occurs when there is a public attempt to share and remains as tacit (inert) knowledge when there is no coach and no dialogue (see Schön, 1987, pp. 299–302).

Equipped with these perspectives we can now turn to section two of this book and consider supervision in the practice setting.

Further reading

Carr, W. (1987). What is an educational practice? *Journal of Philosophy of Education*, **21**, 163–175.

Eraut, M. (1995). Schön shock: a case for reframing reflection-in-action? *Teachers and Teaching: Theory and Practice*, **1**, 9–23.

Fish, D. (1989). *Learning Through Practice in Initial Teacher Training*. Kogan Page . Chapter 4, pp. 58–71.

Mattingly, C. and Fleming, M. (1994). *Clinical Reasoning: Forms of*

Inquiry in a Therapeutic Practice. F. A. Davis and Co. Especially chapter 2 (pp. 22–34).

Russell, T. (1993b). Critical attributes of a reflective teacher: is agreement possible? In *Conceptualizing Reflection in Teacher Development* (J. Calderhead, and P. Gates, eds) pp. 144–153, Falmer Press.

Schön, D. (1987). *Educating the Reflective Practitioner*. Jossey Bass. Chapter 2, pp. 22–40 is the most important follow-up reading for this chapter. It may need several readings.

Van Manen, M. (1995). On the epistemology of reflective practice. *Teachers and Teaching: Theory and Practice*, 1, 9–23.

Part Two

Practice-focused supervision: a quality approach

4

Quality practice:
versions and views of good practice

Introduction

All professions in health care are being required currently to increase the quality of practice, and the role of the supervisor is central to this enterprise. In nursing, the emphasis placed on good practice and on excellence in practice has been highlighted in a range of government documents. Indeed in *A Vision for the Future* (NHSME, 1993) it states that high quality care and research-based good practice are fundamental to the philosophy of nursing, midwifery and health visiting. (There are some problems about this, though, since 'research' here is defined only as positivistic enquiry designed to extend scientific knowledge.)

The concept of good practice and what is therefore meant by excellence in practice as well as what might be meant by a good educator and an effective therapist, need to be considered very carefully by supervisors.

Wilson offers a taxonomy of a good educator and tries to define the qualities involved. His taxonomy is listed under three broad headings: types of understanding; general virtues and qualities; and types of skill (Wilson, 1993, pp. 140–2). In his last category he offers few items because he believes skills to be least important and 'much more tenuously connected to the basic concept' of a good educator since they depend 'on local and mutable conditions'. He concludes that 'the concept of a good teacher is much more closely allied to common sense thinking than to falsely applied types of expertise – either "theoretical" or "behavioural" ' (Wilson, 1993, p. 142). He also explores, in chapter five, the distinction between two questions: (1) is he professionally competent? (the answer being offered in fairly down-to-earth terms involving knowledge of subject, communication skills, good preparation), and (2) does this person's character make him fit to be an educator? He adds: 'nobody, at least on reflection, really believes that effective education can be reduced to a set of skills; it requires certain dispositions of character . . . and must include positive qualities and virtues (Wilson, 1993, p. 113).

Austin and Herbert (1995), too, attempt a taxonomy – this time of the effective therapist. In seeking to stimulate debate about the development and implementation of clinical guidelines in occupational therapy, and in order to warn OTs about the possible culture change which might ensue, they probe concepts like 'clinical guidelines' and 'professional standards', offering the following list of what they regard as the key components of being a good therapist. These are: being client-centred; using holistic approaches; using innovative practices (being free-thinking and imaginative, developing novel approaches); being a reflective practitioner (learning from practice, trusting informed intuition); making therapeutic use of self; using multiple therapeutic approaches; and operating research-based practice. Yet even these – if used in the wrong place at the wrong time – could result in bad rather than good practice.

In fact 'quality' and 'good practice' are problematic notions which are value-based and context specific and thus are rather more difficult notions than is implied in much government and professional literature. In the past, practitioners have frequently judged good practice on the basis of tacit and unexplored standards. Now the present emphasis on value for money and explicit definitions of standards of practice demand that supervisors be explicit in describing the standard against which they are assessing the practitioner's practice.

It should not, however, be assumed that the existence of these explicit standards will make supervision any more objective. Further, supervisors' own practice in their profession will also be open to scrutiny by both students and practitioners who, in order to develop their practice, will need, with the supervisor's help, to discuss practice in an appropriate language and to consider the processes involved in producing, developing and refining it. This highlights the importance of the relationship between practice and education. Indeed in the context of initial teacher education, Alexander suggests that a minimum condition of partnership between schools and Higher Education (HE) ought to be that the partners *each* 'make explicit and argue their particular versions of good practice through to a point of consensus or its nearest approximation' (Alexander, 1990, p. 72).

This matters, he suggests, because it will help to establish a partnership of equals, and will save difficulties later on. In nursing, as in all other health care professions, this situation is equally pertinent, particularly since, in many cases, the divide continues among theorists and practitioners about definitions and interpretations of good practice. Indeed, developing an interpretation of good practice is complicated by the lack of consensus among theorists and practitioners and by the need to respond to demands in government documents about good practice, and/or in those emanating from public and professional bodies.

Chapter 1 established that many supervision issues are valuebased, and a little thought about the different skills and expertise needed in different clinical settings will suggest that it is essentially context specific. Before tackling these matters in detail, it is important to recognize that not one but a number of issues are at stake here, as the following set of questions attempts to reveal.

Some questions related to clarifying the meaning of good practice:

• What are the constituents of good practice?
• In what range of ways might it be analysed?
• Over how many aspects of professionalism should supervisors seek good practice in practitioners?
• How might good practice be determined?
• How might supervisors judge it?
• What would count as evidence?
• In what language might it be useful to discuss good practice?
• What influential views already exist about good practice?
• How might professionals investigate practice?
• How do practitioners see good practice?
• How might these views affect their observations and their practice?
• How might practitioners be drawn to reconsider their views about good practice?

This chapter tackles these questions in three sections as follows: a consideration of some concepts associated with good practice, some current influential versions of good practice, and some assumptions underlying both of these; a consideration of evidence for good practice and how practice might be investigated; practitioners' ideas about good practice and how to help them refine these. Finally, some preliminary ideas about some principles of good practice in supervision are offered as a lead into the following three chapters.

Good practice: definitions and assumptions

What constitutes good practice?

That professional activity which practitioners label as good practice is that which they value. Once again, the overall models of professional practice presented in Chapter 2 serve to help us explore these issues. The following offers two polarized versions of these in order to enable supervisors to explore their own views.

Task 4.1 Points for reflection

Consider the following paragraphs critically and seek as you do so to consider your own views.

Bear in mind the possible distinction between your espoused theories and your theories-in-use (see Chapter 3 for detailed discussion of these concepts).

Those who subscribe to the technical–rational view of practice accept a mastery of skills approach and therefore believe that good practice is about specifying and then mastering the necessary skills to a given, visible and measurable standard. Such skills they see as mainly practice delivery skills. These are often considered to be context specific. This approach is considered to offer an objective means of assessing practitioners' practice, though for some that objectivity is a chimera, being shot through with value judgements at all points. Those who adopt the technical–rational approach seek to establish the specific skills and their specific standards. To achieve this they either emphasize the development of competencies (which may have been identified by non-practitioners), or they use the equally technical–rational approach of employing empirical-analytic models established by research which seeks to develop a deductive system of predicting and controlling the outcome of practice (Acton, Irving and Hopkins, 1991). These versions of the technical–rational approach beg all the questions about the criteria for deciding the skills, about how they can be mastered, how many of them must be mastered to be a good practitioner and what (quantitatively and qualitatively) will count as evidence of that mastery. Indeed the debate over the now 'classical' evidence provided by Benner (1984) in her study on the different levels of competence between novice and expert practitioners demonstrates the different interpretations among nurses as to appropriate knowledge for different levels of practitioners (English, 1993; Darbyshire, 1994). Under this view, then, good practice is achieved as a result of someone outside the profession decreeing a standard and supervisors ensuring its implementation (see Chapter 7). The language in which good practice is discussed under this view is the confident language of the mastery of skills. Bullough and Gitlin describe this problem in initial teacher education by saying that 'the beginning teacher's theories are ignored, or deemed illegitimate or irrelevant to learning to teach' (see Bullough and Gitlin, 1994, p. 70).

Those who subscribe to the professional artistry view eschew the notion that the essence of practice is conveyed in pre-specifiable skills, do not believe that the same agenda of skills is necessary for everyone and reject the idea of mastery of professional practice. This does not mean, however, they pay no attention to skills but that these are discussed in terms of the principles upon which they are based and are attended to as they become significant in the practical setting. Those subscribing to this view consider practice at the level of principle, and seek to place practitioners' development within an educational framework, in order to develop a professional person rather than a skilled practice deliverer. They seek to enable practitioners to establish principled practice, the procedures of which will transcend specific contexts. Their aims, developed from their view of good practice, involve the development of professional insight from intuition, and the ability to exercise practical wisdom and professional judgement so that practitioners know when and how to develop the skills they have learnt. They argue that practice is refined and ideas developed about what is good practice by practising, investigating practice systematically and considering practice in debate with others (clients, colleagues and writers). On this view, standards arise from professional improvement from within, and at the centre of this process is systematic reflection on practice, endemic to which is also a seeking of broader perspectives on practice.

For some, then, striving for good practice is product-centred, i.e. it is about trying to implement predetermined skills. For others it is about processes and principles and involves continual seeking.

Various versions of good practice

The everyday professional life of practitioners is full of both formal and informal occasions on which professionals and non-professionals make judgements about practitioners and practice, e.g. validation and accreditation visits (by universities and professional bodies); interview panels; appraisal interviews; supervision of practice; research reports; consumer groups; community health councils; staff informal talk; patient and client grapevines. Some of these judgements are often made on the basis of very little, if any, empirical evidence. Only the most formal of these occasions ever state the criteria against which such judgements are made, and then those criteria are not always central to the final decisions. Worse, perhaps, a range of *different* criteria can often be operating within one practice setting. Mattingly and Fleming (1994) show how OTs often have to work between two different discourses. They offer us a vivid example of the sort of double bind that OTs can find themselves in (and which we believe in future, if not at present, is as likely to occur in Britain as in America) and illustrate the 'disjunction between what therapists do and what they report to others', as follows:

To be a good professional in the eyes of non-occupational therapy colleagues, and to ensure their services were billable, therapists were driven to narrow the scope of their treatment goals and activities along more biomedical lines – to treat the physical body. But to be a good professional in attending to the meaning of disability and to elicit the strong commitment of clients, therapists were drawn to broaden the scope of clinical problems, addressing many 'real life' issues that did not yield neat, precise or measurable outcomes. Many therapists were masterful in understanding patients and the illness experience...Because they valued this work, they continued with it. But because it was not 'reimbursable', they did not document it. We soon came to call this the 'underground practice' (Mattingly and Fleming, 1994, p. 296).

They concluded that OTs values 'often bring them into conflict (though often a silent conflict) with the values of the dominant bio-medical culture held by other members of the clinical world' (Mattingly and Fleming, 1994, pp. 296–7).

It is thus a major question as to whether specific criteria or rules and procedures set down external to the individual context are ever of any great value in considering good practice and assessing the performance of practitioners, or whether recourse to considering the practitioner's operating principles is more useful.

The technical–rational view of practice, as has been described, embraces inspection and control occasions. For its adherents, objec-tively stated examples of good practice are important. The attempts by the Department of Health in England, by reference to models of good practice, highlight the difficulties of identifying criteria which deter-mine good practice in health care. Indeed in the publication *The A–Z of Quality* (NHSME, 1993a), although a range of good models has been identified there has been no attempt to analyse what it is about these examples of practice which make them 'good practice'. For some exam-ples it is difficult to see why they have been included since they are examples of everyday practice. A similar situation has been reported by Broadhead (1987) in teaching, where an analysis of significant publica-tions from the Department of Education and Science/Her Majesty's Inspectors (DES/HMI) in the late 1970s and the early 1980s failed to identify any reference to a framework of self-improvement, in that the models focused only on the end product of an ideal teacher, and failed to address the detailed complexity of the primary classroom. They also suggest strongly that by acquiring certain behaviours teachers will improve their classroom efficiency (Broadhead, 1987, pp. 68–9). Thus, they are inclined to be stereotypical and ignore the complexity of real classrooms. There are also problems in health care practice, where government documents such as those cited above, identify case studies of individual good practitioners from which they attempt to deduce some rules of good practice to be applied generally, and offer advice that can be distorted by being generalized from the particular and which may be inappropriate if applied to other situations.

Task 4.2 Reflecting on good practice

Identify two key documents in your own profession which seek to define, discuss or impose upon practitioners views about 'good practice'. For each document analyse *critically*, and make notes about:

- the document's aims
- the authors of the document and the body which has published it
- the context out of which it has come (historical, social, political, professional trends)
- the ideas about good practice that it promulgates
- the values, assumptions and beliefs that underlie these
- the influence it has had on practitioners (and on professional bodies/ the public?)

The following two pages offer examples from nursing of the sort of documents that might be chosen.

Targeting Practice: The Contribution of Nurses, Midwives and Health Visitors (DoH, 1993) is an example from nursing of the type of publication described above. This document, produced following the initiative on the *Health of the Nation* (DoH, 1992) was a result of a trawl by the government, in collaboration with professional statutory bodies and professional organizations, to identify examples of good practice. The government, using the services of an external management consultant, collected examples of nursing interventions from a range of clinical settings to provide practitioners with illustrations of good practice. It is interesting that the publication admits that the examples were neither selected nor formally evaluated by the Department (DoH, 1993, p. 2). From their examples the following technical–rational list of good practice in nursing has been identified:

- nurses should play a key role
- practice is based on best research evidence available. (It is disturbing to note that no definition is given as to what is meant by research.)
- practice has clear objectives, targets and standards
- objectives and targets are achievable and consistent with *Health of the Nation* and local targets

- practice is clearly defined and well implemented
- practice is delivered in an environment conducive to the achievement of objectives
- practice has the commitment of everyone including senior managers
- the nurses involved have clear responsibilities and authority
- there is evidence of cost benefit/option appraisal
- practice demonstrates appropriate alliances
- there is evidence of formal evaluation
- the results are widely disseminated
- practice will be acted on (DoH, 1993, p. 8).

This list again suggests that good practice is generalizable, unproblematic and achievable by all. In fact many questions remain, not only about the methods used to generate these particular examples of good practice, but also the extent to which they enable practitioners to interpret and adopt good practice.

Griffiths (1995), in his review of the literature, points out how little progress has been made in identifying clear outcomes of nursing practice and what little research there has been in this area. He goes on to cite standard setting as one methodological approach contributing to the evaluation of outcomes of nursing, which in turn contributes to the identification of good practice. The publication of guidelines for the development of good practice by the Royal College of Nursing in the UK, as part of the Dynamic Quality Improvement Programme, is an illustration of this approach. However, standards are not 'natural phenomena', like mountains, to be found in the world, rather, they are man-made notions and (despite what politicians would have us believe) they have no absolute empirical foundation. In fact the whole process of standard setting is problematic and can be interpreted as a technical–rational approach to practice. As Hartley has shown, this technocratic view of life can be traced back to Bentham whose ideas about 'normalizing judgement' (standardization) have become so commonplace that we are no longer aware of other ways of thinking, but readily accept a view of life in which components, lists and taxonomies are invented to enable those who monitor and measure to pretend they have an absolute against which to judge. As a result of this need, the invention of standards and the measurement of performance both become ends in themselves (Hartley, 1992, pp. 32–7).

Benner (1984), in attempting to identify excellence in practice, does not focus on outcomes of care, but identifies domains and competencies of expert practitioners which were developed from nurses' descriptions of episodes of care. Within each of the seven domains of practice she identifies a set of competencies. Although she states these lists are not exhaustive or even comprehensive, the use of terms such as competencies suggests that despite the possible use of this research in encouraging reflection on practice, this work is still influenced by a technical–rational view of professionalism, which needs to be borne in mind as it is used.

For those who espouse the professional artistry approach, the judgements which are most valuable and often most powerfully influence and refine practice are those made by practitioners about themselves as a result of investigating their actions, and enlightening their findings by reference to the work of others (colleagues/writers). From such investigations principles of procedure can be built. To this end, a vital set of processes in the supervision of practice are the means to investigate personal practice. By using such processes, which include entering into dialogue with the situation and bringing to it critical perspectives from one's own thinking and from the work of others, the professional artist is developed. This process is not specific only to professional development but can be used from the very beginning of professional education as a *modus operandi* built into the very foundation of professional practice. For this reason, the following section looks in some detail at investigating practice. First, however, supervisors may need to review something of their own practice and their views about good practice.

The supervisor's perception of good practice

The majority of supervisors are experienced practitioners with a range of ideas and expertise about what is meant by good professional practice. In addition, many supervisors will be currently involved in practice and there is no doubt that the supervisor will need to be well aware of the strengths and problems of his or her own practice and be able to discuss this with the practitioners they are supervising. Indeed as Wilkin (1992) highlights in the context of the supervision in community psychiatric nursing, the process has a dual role of not only enabling practitioners to improve practice, but also encouraging practitioners to explore areas within themselves which may inhibit the development of excellence in practice. Since caring plays a fundamental role in nursing interventions (Benner and Wrubel, 1989), and in the work of all health care professionals, this situation is equally significant to all professional groups. In addition, as many supervisors continue to have a practice responsibility, these issues are also important to their own clinical practice, and provide them with the opportunity of exploring their own practice interventions in a new light. In this way their own practice provides an important learning opportunity for the practitioners whom they are supervising.

Providing an environment appropriate to supervision requires supervisors to be able to articulate clearly what is involved in their own work, but, for some very good reasons, this has proved difficult. Fish, Twinn and Purr (1990) in a study of reflective practice in the professional preparation of teachers and health visitors demonstrated the difficulty experienced by expert practitioners in articulating their practice. Yet to be able to discuss an episode of practice and to be able to pinpoint those elements in it of good practice and its underlying principles of procedure are basic to the process of supervision. Practitioners need help in seeing and then in identifying what it is they are looking at. Supervisors clearly will need to help supervisees to build up experience of this. To that end Task 4.3 is offered and should be attempted now.

Looking at oneself, one's practice and one's underlying views of good practice (beliefs/assumptions/theories) in this way can be decidedly uncomfortable. As Jennifer Nias points out, it involves seeing oneself anew, and this brings with it additional anxiety and vulnerability (Nias, 1987, p. 13). As Broadhead says in the context of teaching, perception is not just seeing, but involves interpretation, and the ability to distinguish between crucial and less important issues in teaching and learning, and the ability to articulate what is seen (Broadhead, 1990, p. 126). Speaking of using video to capture and investigate one's practice, she points out the 'feelings of dis-equilibrium that viewers of self may experience . . . as they attempt to reconcile what they see of themselves and the impact of their actions on the classroom, with an inner conviction of what they may believe themselves to be doing and the impact they believe it is having' (Broadhead, 1990, p. 127). She also lists seven questions that viewers might ask of their work when it is first videoed, and which teachers preparing to work as mentors and therefore to open their practice to critical scrutiny of others, might also find a useful starting point. These questions adapt well to the health care professions since they are equally relevant to all practitioners responsible for supervision. Broadhead's questions, adapted for the health care professions, are as follows:

- Do I look like the practitioner I think I am?
- Do I look like the person I think I am?
- Am I behaving in ways in which I think I behave?
- Will others see me as I see myself?
- Do I want to modify the image I have of myself?
- How easy will that be?
- What are the implications for my practice? (adapted from Broadhead, 1990, p. 134).

It should also be noted carefully that observable evidence is also liable to misinterpretation since what is visible is often ambiguous and

Task 4.3 Points for action and discussion

Use one side of one piece of A4 for the first three questions.

1 Write down your key views on what is good practice in your clinical area. Take a bit of time on this – don't just dash down the first two things you think of. Imagine that you might be addressing a colleague in preparation for supervising a practitioner.
2 Write down your essential views about patient/client care. (Audience as above.)
3 Write down (briefly!) your *management* structure's* views about patient and client care and the practice to provide that care (what is your *evidence?*)

*If you do not work within the Health Service/private sector, you may need to interpret this phrase in relation to your professional body, or to whatever structure you are answerable to.

4 *On a clean sheet of A4 paper using one side only:*
 Describe in detail as to a colleague from another institution a *small* piece of your own practice (perhaps one episode of care) of which you have recently been particularly proud. Don't get too hung up on explaining the contextual details – say the minimum necessary for an outsider to grasp your main issues. Say *more* about the meat of the good practice. Use points. Tell the story of the episode of care or part of it. Think of your audience as a practitioner who had watched the practice but might not have noticed some aspects.
5 *On a third sheet of A4, using one side only*, say as exactly as possible *why* it was good practice. What was good about it? Explain as to a practitioner the key aspects of its good practice.
6 Share your written responses to 4 with a colleague with whom you don't usually work.
7 Ask the colleague (by deduction) to jot down what seem to be your views on practice in your profession that underlie your description as given in 5 above.
8 Compare what your colleague wrote with your own comments in answer to question 5. Any points additional to your own may show theories/values/beliefs that you were not aware of.

• Any key differences between your answers to questions 1 and 2 and to question 5 may indicate a tension between your beliefs about good practice and your actual practice (your espoused theories and your theories-in-use).
• Equally, it is important to recognize that there is an element of subjectivity in all of this, and that the whole exercise has underlying it views about good practice which need to be further examined.

Task 4.4 Points for action

(We wish to make the point that ethical issues need to be considered in carrying out this task, but that since the intention of this task is to focus on the practitioner not the client or patient, gaining access for the task should not be too difficult.)

1 Set up a video camera in an episode of care which you would like to investigate or ask a colleague to video you. (About 20 minutes is all you want.)
   Or/and on another occasion, set up a tape recorder while you work with patients/clients.
2 Review the tape afterwards in private and with plenty of time to think about it.
3 Ask yourself Broadhead's questions.
4 Recapture if possible what you were thinking as you worked (your reflections-in-action).
5 Ask patients/clients (and any other adult present) what they thought was happening in that episode of care. (These are ways of gaining other perspectives on, and other interpretations of events.)

---

is rarely the whole story. It is usually necessary therefore to consider a range of perspectives in the issue under consideration.

And so we begin to see the need to investigate our practice more systematically. Supervisors will need to discuss with practitioners this approach to developing practice – and even to offer themselves as an example of doing so. The following section offers some perspectives on this.

Good practice: seeking the evidence

Learning good practice: a contribution from research

It is clear then from the above that there are a number of ways in which research knowledge about practice can be harnessed by professionals in pursuit of improving their practice or of achieving good practice. For example, they can use research conducted by others for a variety of purposes, or they can conduct their own investigations. Before the practitioner is able to take advantage of any of these, however, he or she needs to understand how different approaches to research operate. The following two sub-sections attempt to explain the broad differences between the main research approaches, and to offer some ways in which practitioners can investigate their own practice.

Extending understanding or proving the point?

In spite of some recent publications on practitioner research in nursing and health care more generally (Reed and Procter, 1995), there is still among professionals a tendency to equate research with the gathering of large quantities of data in pursuit of proving hypotheses – but this is only one approach to research. It is the scientific domain, world-view or 'paradigm' of research. Its bases are found in scientific approaches. It operates on a large scale and views its findings as hard knowledge which professional practitioners should find their own ways of implementing. Its language is the language of proof and evidence. It seeks to provide a foundation of new knowledge. That is, it seeks truth. It is reductionist in that the scale of its operations requires a recourse to reducing ideas to numbers or models. It claims to be objective. It does not always draw attention to the fact that its findings are themselves only *theories*. For practitioners the advantages of outsider researchers (people whose profession is researching rather than clinical practice) are that they can offer a fresh view of practice. However, it nearly always simplifies the true complexities of the practice setting and, in its processes, results and recommendations, does not always take full account of the real requirements of a practising professional. The technical–rational view tends to look to this sort of research to help in the improvement of practice. But, as authors such as Bond (1993) for nursing, and Reed and Proctor (1995) for the health care professions suggest, the limitation and difficulties of using a positivist approach in nursing research are considerable, particularly if one is seeking an understanding of the complexity of practice. Bond argues that practitioners 'often have to get inside the black box' if an understanding of the complexities of practice intervention is to be achieved (Bond, 1993, p. 100). Benner (1984) argues that 'although theories guide clinicians ... any nurse experienced in working with these theories finds differences that the formal theory fails to express'.

An alternative approach is that of the humanistic, or interpretative paradigm of research. Its bases are found in the social sciences and many of its methods are derived from the arts. It operates on a small scale, and seeks to understand an individual case rather than to prove knowledge on a large scale. That is, it seeks wisdom. This broad approach provides a means for the individual practitioner to find out about and to understand his or her practice better.

Taking an investigative stance to practice

To be a reflective practitioner is to be committed to reflection on and investigation of one's practice in order to refine and improve it continuously. This approach is seen by many as an essential part of quality practice. This means that practice and research are seen as closely interrelated. Indeed, reflection may be both a means of investigating practice and the stimulus for further investigation.

The *audience* for this may be personal. It may be one's colleagues (shared through the clinical setting or professional organization; or used as evidence of one's progress in professional development during appraisal). It may be the wider reading world. By sharing ideas and the fruits of investigation we are all the gainers in improved understanding and perhaps refined practice. Importantly, for the supervisor, the audience may (some might argue 'should') be the practitioner being supervised.

There seems then to be little doubt that investigating one's practice is a natural part of developing practice or at least of being a professional, reflective practitioner. Investigation of one's practice can be on a very small and personal scale and need not take up much time in addition to one's professional engagements. One can take a look at an episode of care and can enlighten, refine and improve practice and re-enliven work that might otherwise become routine. As Rudduck says within the context of teaching:

> After a while, teachers see what they expect to see and constantly reconstruct the classroom in its own image. Reflective research is a way of helping teachers to sharpen their perceptions of the everyday realities of their work; it helps them to identify worthwhile problems to work on, and through their enquiry to extend their understanding, insight and command of the situations in which they work.

This, she argues, enables teachers to see the 'contradictions of purpose and value' in their work, and to monitor whether their strategies achieve their intended purpose. She adds, significantly for supervisors:

> the likelihood of teachers opting to learn from the thoughtful and critical study of their own practice is greater if such activity has been legitimised during initial training (Rudduck, 1992, p. 164).

In nursing, authors such as Benner (1984) and Gray and Forsstrom (1991) argue the significance of reflective processes in the reassessment of nursing interventions and practice. In addition research by Fish, Twinn and Purr (1990) supported the notion of the importance of practitioners developing these processes during their initial preparation for practice. Research in progress may soon offer examples for a range of professions of how health care practitioners have learnt about themselves and their practice by harnessing methods of systematic reflection.

The more difficult question is how best to do this. Some would argue that purely reflective research is enough, some say that critical action research needs to be harnessed to this, some argue for narrative enquiry as an alternative to action research, some prefer the development of small-scale practitioner-focused case study.

Reflective research is a broad term for investigating one's own practice and immediate working arena with a view to improving it as a result of reflecting upon it. Rudduck (1992) argues that it 'is a way of building personal excitement, confidence and insight and these are important foundations for career-long personal and professional development'.

Action research has as its main justification the improvement of practice. It is, as a result, overtly political, and can see reflection as less significant than action, emphasizing the changes to be made to future practice rather more than the understanding of present practice (and in that sense can even be confused with audit – see Bennett, 1994). Lomax (1995) offers six principles that guide her own action research in professional practice (some of which could equally characterize other forms of practitioner research). She argues that action research:

- is about seeking improvement by intervention
- involves the researcher as a main focus of research
- is participatory and involves co-researchers rather than informants
- is a rigorous form of enquiry that leads to the generation of theory from practice
- needs continuous validation by educated witnesses from the context it serves
- is a public form of enquiry.

Some would argue that only the first of these really sets action research apart from case study.

Some action research clearly already offers useful perspectives on practice in health care, and to some extent shows the political characteristics described above. For example, Steward (1994) sought to discover how clinical supervisors, students and their tutors perceived fieldwork associated with an occupational therapy degree course, in order to use this knowledge and institute collaborative action planning in fieldwork education. She also discusses the pleasures and problems of action research. Further, Titchen and Binnie (1993) offer a 'unified action research strategy' for nursing, in which they declare that action research involves five activities: introducing innovation and facilitating change; helping practitioners to research their own practice; facilitating professional learning and reflective practice; working towards democratization of health care through the emancipation of nurses from oppressive hierarchies; and generalizing and testing theory. Sparrow and Robinson (1994), however, raise questions about whether action research is an appropriate design for research in nursing and conclude that it may not be the least problematic nor the most appropriate design for the investigation of nursing. Further, and significantly, they warn that it can be particularly dangerous in the hands of, or commissioned by, managers in the present unstable conditions of the NHS. Landgrebe and Winter (1994) provide insights into the value and implications of reflective writing in action research in relation to carers learning from dying patients. It is, however, doubtful if this is really action research – it seems more like narrative enquiry.

Narrative enquiry is a very useful and fast developing technique in health care. It should be seen in the context of critical appreciation, and involves practitioners in recounting stories about their own practice with a view to understanding it better and refining it. Key proponents of this include: Benner (1984), Darbyshire (1991) and Robb and Murray (1992) in nursing; Mattingly and Fleming (1994) in occupational therapy; Bradley (1992) for general practitioners; Benett and Danczak (1994) who write about the reflections in a primary health care team; and Thow and Murray (1991) in physiotherapy. There are also important examples of the use of autobiography in reflecting on practice in the seminal work of Boud, Keogh and Walker (1985) and Wood (1987).

Case study is a highly useful approach in practitioner research. Indeed, Golby argues that 'case study, properly conceived, is uniquely appropriate as a form of educational research for practitioners to conduct', since it has the potential to 'relate theory and practice, and advance professional knowledge by academic means' (Golby, 1993b, pp. 3–4). He argues that case study is 'not the name of a method but more a signal that a concrete instance is to be investigated' and that the enquirer will use any tools which are appropriate to the question and the situation (see Golby, 1989, p. 168). Case study allows for the study of 'particular incidents and events, and the selective collection of information on biography, personality, intentions and values (which) allows the case study worker to capture and portray those elements of a situation that give it meaning' (Walker, 1986, p. 189). Case study is a systematizing of experience, which has the quality of undeniability. Such studies are 'intensive investigations of single cases which both serve to identify and describe basic phenomena, as well as provide the basis for subsequent development' (Kenny and Grotelleuschen, 1984, p. 37). Case study can be merely descriptive, can be analytical or can be deliberative. As Golby explains, generalization from such study can only be made when the *particular* rather than the unique nature of the study is identified, that is when it is clear 'what the particular case is a case of'. The unique, by its very nature, is unable to be thus classified and it therefore becomes impossible to discuss it in general terms (see especially Fish and Purr, 1991, p. 23; Golby, 1993b, pp. 6–9). Case study can thus, very usefully, provide the data for reflection on detailed practice and its wider implications.

In all research, the aims and the focus of the investigation are the most significant considerations. However, they can sometimes cause the research approach to be unnecessarily limited or misdirected. Just as there can be a simplistic and inward looking version of reflective research which aims only at inert reflection, so, too, there can exist a simplistic version of action research which rushes precipitately into action aimed at change and where there is little overt recognition of some of the more problematic aspects of education and no way of ensuring that the moral and ethical aspects of practice are attended to. Webb (1993), while acknowledging the difficulties, ethical issues and complexities of practitioners using action research in the practice setting, highlights the richness of experience and data which result from this approach, particularly in initiating and evaluating innovations in practice. Narrative enquiry as a research approach needs more development and acknowledgement in its own right in health care so that it is not simply used as a springboard for or starting point in other kinds of research. Case study which is sometimes wrongly confused with 'taking a case', is arguably the most open approach and is the most easily operated by an individual practitioner enquirer.

There is evidence then that it is possible for practitioners to take on a research/inquiry dimension in their clinical setting, via reflective research, critical action research, narrative enquiry, or – perhaps particularly – case study, and that the activities of reflection, of producing narratives of episodes of care and case studies, can provide a language in which to discuss practice and its development. Readers are directed to the extensive literature on enquiry methods in qualitative research if they wish to pursue these matters further.

It is important to remember, though, that practitioners bring their own knowledge to the supervision process. Included in that knowledge are their own views about good practice, which obviously must be considered within that process.

Good practice: practitioners' views

Informed understanding or unquestioned assumptions?

Although there will be some practitioners who come to the supervision process with many years of experience, all practitioners with whom supervisors have contact will have had some experience of practice and these experiences will have not only informed their understanding of practice but also their interpretation of good practice. However, their interpretation of good practice may be open to challenge, as well as raising important implications for the supervision process. As authors such as Walsh and Ford (1989) demonstrate, many practitioners continue to use tradition and myths to inform patient and client care despite a growing body of nursing research. Indeed in their more recent publication they raise questions about new rituals substituting those of old, as practitioners adopt new approaches to practice with little attempt to evaluate or critique that approach to patient or client care (Ford and Walsh, 1994). Such experiences, which practitioners bring with them to the supervisory process, have significant implications for the supervisor.

How supervisors work on these views of practice

Supervisors therefore need to acknowledge and work with the different views of good practice that practitioners bring to the supervision session. Johns (1993) provides an illustration of one way of working with practitioners using the process of reflection to guide the supervision session. An important focus in this approach is not only the use of a reflective diary from which the supervisee selects experiences which he or she is comfortable to share with the supervisor, but also the use of note taking by the supervisor to ensure continuity of the process and to validate the interpretation of the discussion that has taken place in previous supervision sessions. The supervisor also plays an important role in using relevant theory to match experiences emerging from the discussion between the supervisor and practitioner. This process allows practitioners to explore their perceptions of that clinical experience as well as articulate their experiences in practice. The use of this approach allows supervisors to debate and understand the underlying beliefs and assumptions of the practitioner. By this means the practitioner's tacit views about good practice are made explicit. These views are then open to public discussion and thus to reconsideration and to challenge. The supervisor's task here is to ensure that practitioners become aware of alternatives, and that they also begin to recognize that uncertainty and the admission of ignorance are the means to developing practice. This process can, of course, be painful, but without it little progress can be made in learning through practice. Time is needed for this to have effect and for revisiting the crudity of the emerging notions. Direct challenge is not always helpful at this point. Neither is offence at student critique. Discussion needs to be managed by someone who does not feel challenged personally by practitioners' comments and who enables the students to work through their views and to see for themselves the need to modify them. This, then, is yet another dimension of enabling practitioners to develop their practice, but it requires distance in space and time from the practice setting, and for many practitioners and supervisors this may be difficult to create, which highlights another of the complex issues involved in good practice in supervision.

Good practice in supervision

Generally, practitioners will consider supervisors to have a wide range of knowledge which will help them develop their practice, but there is often a lack of understanding on the part of both practitioners and supervisors about how practitioners might gain access to such knowledge. This is because we are now so conditioned by the 'delivery' metaphor to think of teaching as 'giving to others', that the key notion of facilitating practitioners to learn for themselves easily slips out of our sight. If, however, the processes of learning through practice as described in Chapter 3 have anything to teach us about good supervision practices, it is, arguably, that facilitating learning is a vital approach for the supervisor. Readers are now invited to consider critically the following suggested principles of good supervision practice.

- A supervisor is a facilitator who empowers practitioners and draws them to learn for themselves by reflecting on practices.
- The supervisor is not an expert 'knower'. Practitioners already have much knowledge and some may need to be jolted out of being authority dependent. They need to recognize what they know and can do and which parts of their work need developing or refining.
- Supervisors need the skills, abilities and capacity to enable practitioners to develop through practice, and to (re)construct their own knowledge for themselves and each other by deliberating together. Supervisors need to be able to set the atmosphere for this and to establish norms and modes of operation that foster that sort of professional development.
- Supervision is about helping practitioners to question the taken-for-granted, and to see things anew – even to go on wondering/worrying at issues long after the session.
- Disagreements (impersonal ones) are a major means of learning. Passion can get in the way. Supervisors need to keep the balance between objectivity and passion.
- Evidence and reasoning are vital in enabling practitioners to recognize their values/beliefs – reconsider them – perhaps 'know them for the first time' and *then* decide what to do about them. Supervisors need to discipline the debate and order the processes.

- It is very important for the supervisor to create a climate in which it is safe for practitioners to develop and to bare their real views, ideas, beliefs, and also their errors, and problems (which are the learning points of practice).
- Supervisors need to establish the fact that ambiguity and uncertainty are the important norms. Practitioners need to see that 'knowing for sure' is suspect in developing professional practice.
- The agenda needs to include inquiry into everything. A supervisor's role is to be an example of an inquiring and reflective practitioner – to be prepared to be made the *subject* of inquiry by developing practitioners!
- A supervisor's role is to support while also challenging. Challenge should not be destructive. A supervisor therefore needs to understand and be comfortable with both these issues and these processes.
- A supervisor's practice should show that professional development makes one less certain, not more. Learning is about saying 'I think X', not: 'You should think X' or 'I know X'. Supervision is not about telling the practitioner.
- Supervisors need to be able to be challenged and look deeply at their own practice and have disagreements about it without getting personally or emotionally thrown. Looking in depth at even a small piece of one's practice can be very alarming.
- Supervisors need to be able to help practitioners to respond positively to challenge and support them in this and know how to handle the issues about evidence.
- A supervisor's evaluation of a practitioner's performance should show evidence of the important kinds of learning and development described above, and not only be focused on clinical skills.

The reader might wish to use these views to define his or her own philosophy of supervision. The following chapters also seek to provide a practical base for doing this.

Further reading

Alexander, R. (1990). Partnership in initial teacher education: confronting the issues. In *Partnership in Initial Teacher Training* (M. Booth, J. Furlong and M. Wilkin, eds) pp. 59–73, Cassell.

Anning, A. *et al.* (1990). *Using Video-recording for Teacher Professional Development*. University of Leeds School of Education.

Bell, J. *et al.* (1984). *Conducting Small-scale Investigations in Educational Management*. Harper and Row.

Hopkins, D. (1985). *A Teacher's Guide to Classroom Research*. Open University Press.

Kyriacou, C. (1993). Research on the development of expertise in classroom teaching during initial teacher training and the first year of teaching. *Educational Review*, **45**, 78–88.

Nias, J. (1987). *Seeing Anew: Teachers' Theories of Action*. Deakin University.

Reed, J. and Proctor, S. (eds) (1995). *Practitioner Research in Health Care: the Inside Story*. Chapman and Hall.

5

Observing students and being observed

Introduction

The role of direct observation of practice is well established in many health care professions, although in nursing, where much supervision is based on reported practice, particularly in the supervision of qualified practitioners, it is less so. Obviously in some caring situations, those that are of a particular intimate or sensitive nature, the presence of a third person may affect the quality of care offered to the client. However, it is also frequently this type of situation which is the most complex and demanding for practitioners which demonstrates the importance of receiving feedback on directly observed practice. The research by White *et al.* (1994) illustrates the difficulties of students not being directly observed in practice and the implications this has for the opportunity for reflection on practice and maximizing professional development. Thus, although there are difficulties in operating direct observation in health care practice, we believe that this process makes a crucial contribution to the development of professional practice and should be used whenever possible.

The process of observation can be used in one of three ways. First the practitioner or student may observe the supervisor. Secondly the supervisor may observe the student or practitioner and finally both the supervisor and the student together may observe another practitioner. In addition, the use of video allows both practitioners and students to observe their own practice. Although observation is an essential process in facilitating learning and professional development, if it is used inappropriately, without a clear purpose, and in ignorance of its nature and its potential as an approach to finding out about practice, it can provide a thoroughly unhelpful experience not only for students and practitioners but also for supervisors.

Observation is a research technique, and there are a number of investigative tools associated with it, each of which is a specialist implement. It is the nature of observation to concentrate only on the known and visible aspects of a performance. Some of the most important aspects of high quality care and the fostering of this by practitioners are not easily seen. The smooth surface of good practice often renders them invisible. Equally, the surface failure of a particular episode of practice does not necessarily mean that the practitioner is a failure. Thus when, how and why to employ observation (as an approach to enabling students and practitioners to learn or develop their practice), and what it can and cannot tell one about practice, all need to be carefully considered by the supervisor.

This chapter seeks to enable supervisors to think about some useful principles of observation in clinical practice and suggests some tasks which will enable them to investigate these principles further. It considers the nature of observation and focuses on the supervisor operating as observer of the student or practitioner and on the student or practitioner observing the supervisor. In either case the overall intention of most observation is to enable meaning to emerge from the experience, just as was attempted in Chapter 3. It should be noted that the post-practice discussion (known as follow-up or debriefing) is a vital aspect of this whole process. But in order to treat this in detail it has been reserved until the following chapter.

Observation and clinical supervision: an overview

The nature and uses of observation in clinical supervision

As we have said, there are practice situations in which either the dynamics between the patient and client make observation difficult, or in which the caring process may be adversely influenced by the presence of an observer. It is acknowledged that in these situations, direct observation may not facilitate the development of professional practice. Equally, neither will observation benefit the practitioner's development if he or she has not been adequately prepared before the observation session and/or has no opportunity for follow-up afterwards. This section attempts to delineate some of the likely issues about observation which supervisors will need to consider in planning an observation.

The roles of observation in clinical supervision

Observation of practitioners is used for a range of reasons in clinical supervision. It is perhaps a pity that, because the use made of observation in the assessment of clinical practice and its results can thus affect the future of practitioners, many of the occasions on which practice observation occurs are associated with making momentous judgements about practitioners' careers. By contrast, observation of practice is perhaps at its most useful when used as an approach to help practitioners and students to *learn* about and to refine their practice. To be useful in this way to practitioners, the role of observation in supervision needs to be known about and understood by both parties.

This can best be achieved if thought has been given to the range of activities that either improve practice or will help the student make the transition from the relative safety of the practicum to the reality of the practice world. Cameron-Jones (1991) offers a broad framework for drawing a student to learn to teach, which appears equally appropriate to clinical supervision and may help to set observation in context. She discusses what she calls 'thought-oriented methods' where practical matters are aimed at provoking thinking (like explaining, exploring or discussing the traditions of the profession; using a teacher as a model to consider aspects of teaching; discussing case studies; filling in or altering scripts of incidents; and posing dilemmas). These she distinguishes from methods that involve the student in teaching. Here she points to methods that can engage the student gradually in the *practice* of teaching (like isolating a particular skill, strategy or style of teaching; peer teaching; and setting up paired teaching). In fact, quality supervision in clinical practice also utilizes all these techniques. Nevertheless, many of the things that students need to learn cannot be pinpointed by observation alone. It is often necessary to combine observation with interviews or discussion in order to reach the more invisible aspects of practice. Thus, observation is *one* of the methods of finding out about practice.

The importance of purpose in observation

Following Cameron-Jones' classification of different ways of learning about practice, it is important that observation can contribute to a range of purposes, provoking students to think or prompting them to act, as well as being a means of collecting evidence for judgements to be made. Thus, whenever it is used, its purposes must be carefully defined. As Haggar, Burn and McIntyre point out, 'unfocused observation, without a clear purpose is generally demoralising and counter-productive' (Haggar, Burn and McIntyre, 1993, p. 26).

Once the overall purpose is clear then, the focus for the observation, the specific tools for observing, the methods of recording and the ways in which this whole process might be learnt from can all be decided. But though very useful, these tools are also highly dangerous and they need to be employed in the fullest possible knowledge of their strengths and weaknesses. The following section looks at the detail of this.

Techniques for observing and their strengths and weaknesses

Many books on investigating professional practice in health care offer details about practice observation (see, for example, Abbott and Sapsford, 1992). The following can only offer an overview. The techniques and strategies used will need to be appropriate to the focus of the observation. This will depend upon what these strategies can and cannot achieve. What is observed can be narrow or wide in focus. How it is observed will depend upon the overall purpose for the observation. The following represent the major techniques. Some of them emphasize the quantitative approach and seek to reduce what is observed to numbers, some emphasize the qualitative approach which attempts to recognize and preserve the rich complexity of human situations. Proponents of the quantitative approach claim objectivity for it, but in fact this is spurious since subjective judgements are being made at all points in classifying information.

It is possible to take an unstructured approach to observation. That is, it is possible to observe in a naturalistic way without predetermined categories (to watch with an open mind and see what happens). While enabling the observer to see what happens it can also cause failure to notice some quantitative details. It is often used as a first step to narrowing down an observation focus or a research question and can be a useful means of learning about the individual as a practitioner generally.

It is possible to observe using schedules and checklists. In this case, the categories need to be clear. Categories help observers to see some things but blind them to those they have not predetermined. It is regarded as objective, though, as noted above this is not the case. Too many categories can make an observation schedule impossible to use in practice.

It is possible to use a ratings approach. Here a coded scale is set up and the observer rates the occurrence of a particular behaviour, using graphic, numerical or categorical rating scales. The emphasis here is on the number of times a category occurs. Like the checklist approach, it is regarded as objective, though of course judgements are being made each time something is categorized. It is also blinkered and can blind the observer to other issues, particularly where the observer has a limited agenda as to what he or she understands by 'good' practice (Twinn, 1989).

Another dimension that should be considered in observation is the role of the observer in the practice being observed. In participant observation the observer is a normal member of the group, joins in wholeheartedly with the activities, events, behaviours and culture of the group and may not even be known as an observer/investigator or supervisor by the group. The investigator here gains meaning through personal participation. It is not observation alone that informs his or her understanding of the action. This approach offers a better grasp of the complexities of the situation, but it is clearly very subjective and the observer can affect the very practice he or she is observing.

In non-participant observation the investigator is unobtrusive, does not engage in the work of the group as a group member, but remains aloof and distanced from the action. He or she certainly does not feign membership of the group. The observation here is concerned only with participants' behaviours. The focus is on valid recording of behaviours using an unobtrusive strategy of data collection, so as not to interfere with the natural sequence of events. Care is taken not to disturb the ethos and culture of the setting. Yet only the visible is recorded.

It is quite possible to use (in a thoughtful, informed and systematic way) a mixture of these versions. It is also important to think about how they might be supplemented by procedures that will provide complementary data, like interviews, tape-recording of an episode of practice, video camera, stop-frame photography, documentary analysis. Being systematic is important. But the observer always needs to have thought through the strengths, weaknesses and specific possibilities of the approach being used. Account also needs to be taken of the kind of data that will be generated by the chosen techniques, how this will be captured (recorded) and how it will be used in the post-practice discussion.

Some problematic issues

While much of the above seems to suggest that issues in observation are cut and dried, there are many aspects of observation which are problematic. For example, there is no such thing as purely objective, factual observation. All seeing is selective, and all reporting of what is seen is interpretative. Thus, in all observations the 'facts' are coloured by at least two filters. This is true whatever method of observing and recording is adopted. For example, even an observer who seeks and notes down specific instances of a particular behaviour on a checklist (which might seem to be a matter of recording pure facts) is actually interpreting behaviours before deciding which can be counted as specific behaviours to be recorded. And when he or she categorizes them fairly crudely on paper, he or she will also be ignoring other aspects of the practice setting which might have cast a different light on what is being observed. Equally, observers who record in words rather than figures will inevitably indicate some kind of judgement of the situation observed in their choice of expression. Further, with such human and variable activities as nursing and caring in particular, there are likely to be many possible interpretations of most events and the best that an observer can do is to seek several differing perspectives on the event and a range of possible interpretations of it. Task 5.1 will enable readers to investigate this for themselves. Although this task once again requires the use of video, therefore raising possible difficulties for patient and client care, the process will provide valuable learning experiences in developing the skills of the supervisor.

Task 5.1 Points for investigation

1 Video or tape-record about 15 minutes of an episode of practice – yours or a colleague's.
2 Invite several colleagues (or students) without any discussion of the practice beforehand, to watch the video through *once only* and as they watch (and for a few minutes afterwards) to write a clear, simple description of exactly what was happening in the first 10–15 minutes. The practitioner involved in the practice should also do this.
3 Compare what each observer has written (exclude the practitioner involved in the practice from this exercise).
4 Look in detail at the differences between narratives and try to decide why people have written different things – go back to replay the video if you wish to at this point.
5 Compare what observers thought with what the practitioner thought was happening.
6 If you have the chance, find out how the patient/client saw that 15 minutes of the episode of practice.
7 What have you learnt about observation?

What we can now say, then, is that the observer deals not in simple facts but in a version or versions of these. Some useful distinctions are those between analysis (the atomizing of what is seen into its component parts); interpretation (a version or versions of and response to what has been seen from a particular point or points of view); and an appreciation of what has been observed (an artistic critique of what has been seen which offers a view of its successes and failures).

One further matter relates to these issues. As previously described in Chapter 3, unearthing the theories-in-use in practice is a useful means of understanding how a student (or practitioner) thinks and of seeing what informs their professional judgements. It is also important for the observer to be aware of the theories-in-use (both those about practice and those about observation) that direct his or her observation, in order to take account of these and try to keep some balanced judgement about the practice observed. (This is especially important if, for example, the observer is watching activities that run contrary to his or her own preferred way of practising.)

Finally, it is also important to be aware of the complex nature of

---

Task 5.2 Points for investigation

Return to the previous task and ask yourself:

- what theories-in-use directed the practitioner's activities?
- what theories-in-use shaped the observations and interpretations offered?
- what does this reveal about observation?

---

evidence – both what counts as evidence during observation and what it might be evidence of. In the technical–rational view of professionalism, the evidence sought by an observer is that recorded behaviour which will *prove correct* the judgements that have been made. There are problems here however, in that (because of the lack of objectivity in observation) it is difficult to know what some behaviours are evidence of, and it is difficult to be sure how often a behaviour should occur before it can be regarded as definitely evidence of a particular judgement. The professional artistry approach renders this less of a problem since the observer here will seek out critical incidents in the practice observed and then consult the views and understanding of the observed in order to disentangle what rationale actually informed the action. Here, the recorded observations offer the basis for discussion rather than providing evidence in terms of proof, and the reasons for the observer's judgements then spring from the ideas as well as the actions of the practitioner observed.

Equipped with these general principles and issues, it is important to consider the two main aspects of observation, the supervisor being observed and then the supervisor observing. As we have said earlier, although this process is less likely to occur in the supervision of qualified practitioners, it is an invaluable strategy in facilitating quality clinical supervision. In our view therefore, the following strategies are equally appropriate to the process of supervision for both students and practitioners.

The supervisor being observed

The dangers

The beginning of a course of preparation for work in the caring professions usually includes opportunities for the student to think about his or her own practice by means of observing a variety of practitioners at work. Some of those observed will be staff with whom the student otherwise rarely works. All, however, have responsibilities for making the observation an educational experience. This is why such observations need to focus not on how to reproduce the practice observed, but on using what is seen as a means for the student to consider his or her own preferred approaches. But in order to do so, supervisors need to be aware that students can find observation unhelpful as a result of the following conditions:

- The experienced professional being watched is so fluent that it looks easy and no one helps them to see underneath the performance to the expertise. (The practitioner's skill here is often in expert information-processing and speedy decision-making that he or she is hardly aware of him or herself!)
- Students see only what they understand already. They certainly do not understand generally the complexity of practice. The practitioner needs to be articulate about its complexity, and to be able to talk with the student about the issues related to 'good practice'.
- Students often have strong preconceptions about what sort of practitioners they want to be. They are quick to judge those practitioners whom they think are falling short of these preconceptions, and therefore to think that they have little to learn from them.
- Students are generally keen to prove themselves as practitioners. They are eager to get on and learn from their own practice rather than learning from others. (Adapted, with acknowledgement, from Haggar, Burn and McIntyre, 1993.)

Clarifying the purpose of observation

We have already said that having a clear purpose for observation is vital to its usefulness. Within the context of clinical supervision there is a range of purposes for involving students in observing experienced practitioners. Students need to understand in advance of observing: the practitioner's intentions for the episode of care; the context of the observation; and the learning intentions of the observation itself for the student-observer. The student will only really learn from the observation where the supervisor follows it up with the student, both in an open way and by ensuring that predetermined issues have been discussed. Thus, supervisors need to work with the student in discussing the purpose, deciding the focus of the observation, understanding the context, showing the student how to observe and record and in helping the student to use and learn from interpretation, analysis and appreciation of what happened. The following reasons for observing experienced practitioners have been adapted from the work of Haggar, Burn and McIntyre (1993). The explanations below each item are a summary of their ideas.

1 It helps students understand the complexity of practice at the beginning of a course

In order to recognize how much they have to learn, students need to see a range of practice situations, including those of a complex nature, and to hear practitioners *analysing* their own less-than-perfect practice, and considering alternative methods. They need to consider questions like: What would I do now? What are the alternatives? What might the consequences be? What is difficult here? Why?

2 It helps them to learn to analyse what is happening during practice situations

By analysing and interpreting practice in detail they can learn new ways of thinking about incidents in practice and new language and ideas. They need help in learning to see, some simple observation techniques, and discussion before and afterwards. After some practice in analysing strategies in other peoples' practice, they can try them in their own.

3 It offers a sense of the standards practitioners set

Learning what is appropriate when, is difficult. Appropriate practice extends not only to practitioners' interactions with different patients and clients, but also to how they carry out strategies in different practice settings. Professional judgement involves practitioners in making decisions about the appropriateness of care and students need to learn the strategies that practitioners use in making these decisions. Students need to think about their own practice, and how it relates to what they have observed.

4 It shows them different ways of doing things

The focus here is usually strategies in practice. The follow-up needs to highlight things done and their appropriateness; the decisions made as a result of the unexpected; and the ways in which the student can try these things out.

5 It helps them to acknowledge the uniqueness of each practice situation

This can bring home the importance of pacing/timing/need for flexibility, need for responding to individual needs.

6 It helps them identify things they do not understand and which can provide a basis for discussion with the practitioner following completion of the observation session

Here the emphasis will be on the student to raise questions. Indeed students can be educated to raise useful questions in the debriefing, that help them make sense of what they see and help practitioners articulate what they have thought and done. Such questions include:

- How did you achieve . . .?
- Could you explain why . . .?
- What did you do in order to . . .?
- Could you tell me more about . . .?
- How did you know when to . . .?

Haggar, Burn and McIntyre argue that a successful discussion following observation is one where the practitioner does most of the talking and explains the actions he or she has taken, with the discussion revolving around the practice that has been observed. They suggest that by using this approach students learn much more than could be gained just from observation (Haggar, Burn and McIntyre, 1993, handout 4).

Being observed: how will supervisors react?

Being observed is always a slightly uncomfortable experience, even when the observer has been engaged by the person to be observed and the specific purpose and focus has been agreed together as essentially a learning experience rather than an assessment. Under any other circumstances it is even less enjoyable and more judgemental. It can also tempt the person observed into offering an elaborate performance or demonstration which is more for the benefit of the observer than the patient or client. Equally, the observer, by indicating reaction to events, can seriously affect the person observed, while unsympathetic body language from the observer can undermine even the most successful and confident of practitioners. Again, the theories-in-use brought by students in particular to the observation of practitioners can mean that students may have a very distorted view of events, ideas and intentions. It is also clear that in post-practice discussions some students will voice ill-informed judgements about the practice they have observed. Mostly this will be the result of ignorance rather than malice but, unless supervisors take steps to ensure that students are versed in the kinds of positive questions to ask at this point (see above), it can provide practitioners with frustrating situations. Please turn now to Task 5.3 overleaf.

The supervisor observing the student or practitioner

Following the discussion above it is now possible to summarize all that has been said and apply it to the supervisor's observations of the student.

Task 5.3 Points for investigation

1 Ask a colleague to come and observe a small episode of your own professional practice. (Choose a situation you want to find out about and negotiate a clear purpose and focus with the observer.)
2 Ask the observer to be sure to make some written notes during your practice.
3 After the observation, but *before* you discuss together what the observer has to share with you, write down a brief chronological narrative about your own feelings about being observed.
4 What differences did being observed make to your planning; your performance; your interaction with the patient or client?
5 What will you want to tell the observer, to supplement what was visible, in order that the observer better understands your practice and your rationale for action?
6 Now discuss the observer's findings, respond to any questions and then share with him or her your answers to the above.
7 What have you learnt about being observed as a result of this?
8 How will your understanding affect the next occasion on which you are observed by a student or practitioner?
9 How will it affect the next occasion on which you observe a student or practitioner?

The importance of preparation

Overall, then, both observation as an approach, and its specific tools, need to be used as a part of a carefully considered and negotiated programme designed to aid consideration of the complex nature of professional practice as well as to capture aspects of practical activities and seek to improve them. Observation only tells the supervisor so much. Other data collection methods are needed to supplement it. It is behaviour oriented, but this does not always reveal thoughts and intentions. Careful preparation needs to be carried out by observer and observed *together*. Before being observed in practice the student needs to have had a chance to become familiar with the practice situation and to have tried out some of the approaches to be observed. Whether supervisor or student is observed, the intentions of practice need to have been talked through and the observer needs to understand how the observed practice fits within the context of the practice setting. The purpose of the observation, the focus for the observer, the time and place for the post-practice discussion and the rough agenda for it also need to have been agreed. Decisions about all these will depend upon the purposes and focus for the observation, its place in the student's programme, the needs of the patient or client and the student's confidence. Obviously it is important that the relationship between the supervisor and the person being observed is identified, as well as both parties being clear about the purpose of the observation exercise. This is particularly significant if using observation strategies with qualified practitioners where other issues could enter the agenda and confuse the purpose of the observation.

Planning the practical session and the observation

To understand the intentions of practice is to understand much about practice strategies (see Clark, 1988, p. 7). During preparation for the observation session clear agreement/understanding about the following need to be established:

- the overall purposes and the specific purposes for observation
- how these purposes relate to the rest of the student's programme or the professional development of the qualified practitioner
- the specific focus for the observation
- the appropriate observation procedures and strategies to be used
- their strengths and weaknesses
- what will be recorded and how
- how that record will be used
- when and where to discuss the practice afterwards
- in what sorts of terms it will be discussed.

Being in the practice setting

Supervisors need to consider the following about the observation itself:

- how and when to enter the practice setting (should the supervisor be there right from the start?)
- where the supervisor will position him or herself in order to be least obvious to the student or practitioner
- in what frame of mind the supervisor will be watching (with a positive mind-set? will the supervisor be willing to accept different ways of working from his or her own?)
- what will be the relationship of the supervisor with the student or practitioner and the patient or client (how will the patient or client know how to relate to the supervisor)?
- in what ways the supervisor will operate during the episode of practice (will he or she move round or stay still, or interact with the patient or client?)
- how the supervisor will balance observing and recording during the practice.

Supervisors will also need to consider whether they wish to check out other data than that which they can observe passively. It is important to ensure that any incident which disturbs the supervisor during the observation does not colour the overall judgement of the practice – particularly if the student or practitioner adopts a method of practice with which the supervisor is not familiar or does not agree.

Recording observations and use of the records

The importance of recording data during practice observation is paramount. Some observation techniques carry with them a clear indication of how they record data. For example, the checklist approach usually has the items to be observed down the page with the number of occasions observed across it and the ratings approach operates by recording the timing against the categories. In these cases the observer leaves the scene with only maps, ticks on sheets, or figures, all of which rapidly become meaningless once the context has been lost, and none of which offers very firm evidence once the meaning of the categories or the judgements of the observer in respect of the categories is challenged. What is lost is the rich texture of the human interaction. This also means that there is little to be gained by the student at the level of the quality of his or her work.

On the other hand, the unstructured, naturalistic approach can leave the observer unclear what to capture. Here a timed diary is often useful and, of course, tape-recordings offer a further means of capturing the texture of the interaction. Here it is possible, afterwards, to share with the student or practitioner a great deal of evidence, the very nature of which can often also prompt him or her to recall what he or she was thinking or why he or she did or said something and thus to unearth the bases of the professional judgements made.

One of the most useful techniques for getting to the heart of students' or practitioners' professional judgements is to focus on their reflection-in-action. This can be used either generally in considering the observed practice or specifically in looking at a critical incident within it. This involves, *while observing*:

- writing only briefly about what seems to be happening
- simultaneously considering a range of possible explanations for what is happening
- seeking further perspectives on these reasons from within the practice setting (by looking at patients'/clients' care plans or records, asking patients or clients a few questions, looking at resources available

- and, in the light of these, generating in the observation notes a set of questions which will, in discussion afterwards, raise with the student or practitioner some differing explanations for events and responses, and some possible rationales which might underlie actions.

Some of these ideas are akin to the strategies for coaching suggested by Schön (see page 84 above). During the post-practice discussion the student's or practitioner's views about the practical and moral aspects of these can then be sought and, if there is less time than expected for that discussion, the student or practitioner still has access to the notes themselves which will enable him or her to go on thinking about (and even writing about) these matters. Task 5.4 seeks to offer experience of this.

Task 5.4 Points for action

1 Negotiate with a student to observe an episode of his or her practice; clarify the purpose as trying to investigate both his or her reflection-in-action and your skills as a supervisor; clarify the focus of your observation as being a small part of that episode (15 or so minutes will be sufficient).
2 Observe as arranged, noting briefly on a time diary layout the main strategies of practice.
3 Choose two or three key critical incidents where some action and response from the practitioner and/or patient or client was noteworthy in some way, and focus on these, leaving the rest of the practice to continue without your detailed attention (though you should stay in the practice setting).
4 Think about the possible interpretations/explanations/rationales for what happened.
5 Consider whether you can collect any further perspectives on these events (as indicated above) and if so, do so.
6 Try writing down some questions that will unearth these different ways of seeing the events and that will lead the student or practitioner to consider the practical and theoretical aspects of them (including the moral dimensions).
7 Raise these with the student or practitioner after the practice episode.
8 Consider what *you* have learnt as a result of this.

All of this makes for a very useful discussion of qualitative matters, but of course, it prompts questions about debriefing, to which we must now turn. First, however, the following is offered as a framework to help supervisors to consider in detail their work in observing a student or practitioner.

A framework for reflection on observation of practice

Task 5.5 offers a framework for the supervisor who has worked with a student or practitioner in preparing for, carrying out and debriefing an observation, to enable him or her to review and reflect upon practice.

Task 5.5 Reflecting on practice observation

A Purpose of observation
1 What exactly was the purpose of your observation? (Did you have a clear intention?)
2 Was this intention clear to the student or practitioner? (How much of it did that person shape?)
3 What exactly did you intend to focus on during the practice session in order to achieve that purpose?
4 Did you in fact focus on this? (If not, what did you do?)

B Preparation
1 Had you discussed the practice strategy with the student/practitioner prior to the observation?
2 Did you look at the patient's or client's record/notes before the observation? (Were these significant?)
3 What were the student's or practitioner's intentions for the outcome of practice?
4 What preparations had you made for the observation? (Were these sufficient?)

C Evidence
1 What did you set out to watch for and why?
2 How long were you intending to observe for? (Did you? If not, why not?)
3 What *sort* of evidence or information were you collecting?
4 How were you going to use it?
5 How much evidence/information was necessary before you were sure you could come to conclusions?
6 How were you looking? (Wide focus? specific? checklist?)
7 Were you well positioned to see and hear the practitioner and patient/client? (What would have been better?)
8 How did you record your observation? (What was the *format* of your field notes?)
9 How useful were these in your final conclusions?

D Drawing conclusions
1 How have you responded to what happened during the observed practice? Have you utilized a range of analysis, interpretation and appreciation?
2 How have you used your evidence during this process?

---

3 How have the student's/practitioner's comments before and after the observed practice affected your conclusions? (Why?)

4 What other interpretations might have been offered by other colleagues/patients/clients/carers? (How, if at all, might other valid views about 'good practice' have changed the overall conclusions about this practice?)

5 How have you distinguished between what the student/practitioner intended/did and what you yourself would have intended/done in this situation?

6 How have you distinguished between *fact* and *opinion* and recognized the relationship between observation and interpretation?

7 Against what standard were you observing?

8 Were you considering achievement/potential/both? (If both, how?)

9 What allowance did you make for the effect of your presence on the proceedings?

10 What else might you have taken account of before coming to conclusions?

11 Might you have been over-influenced by an incident/aspect of the observed practice?

12 What have you used in evidence for your *final* conclusions?

13 Are you confident that you are using this evidence reasonably, honestly and validly?

E Assessing the observation

1 What theories/beliefs/philosophies/ideas/values/views on 'good practice' influenced the student/practitioner in his or her practice?

2 What theories/beliefs/philosophies/ideas/values/views on 'good practice' influenced your observation of the student's/practitioner's practice?

3 What would you say about the quality of your observation? (Why?)

4 What will you do differently another time? What will you investigate another time?

Further reading

Hopkins, D. (1985). *A Teacher's Guide to Classroom Research*. Open University Press.

Walker, R. (1985). *Doing Classroom Research: a Handbook for Teachers*. Methuen.

Wragg, E. C. (1993). *Classroom Observation*. Cassell.

6
Debriefing, feedback, critique and reflection

Introduction

The use of informed discussion following practice experience is central and essential in helping both students and practitioners to gain access to their practice, and includes consideration of both their performance and their clinical decision-making with all the emotional and moral dimensions that lie under them (see Mattingly and Fleming, 1994). It is this process that enables them to learn, and to develop practice. Indeed the emphasis placed by authors such as White and Ewan (1991) on the processes of debriefing in clinical teaching highlights the significance of this activity in clinical supervision. Yet in many (newer) health care professions the courses of professional preparation being developed still do not give detailed attention to this matter. Although acknowledged as an important role of the supervisor, helping students to learn through their practice is a complex activity that supervisors frequently do not find easy (Twinn, 1992; Fish, Twinn and Purr, 1991). Current models of supervision are often very heavily guided and supervisor dominated (Johns, 1993, 1994). This chapter, therefore, in keeping with the professional artistry approach, attempts to provide supervisors with some *frameworks* to facilitate their work in this role.

First of all, however, the terms must be clarified. The state of the very language in which practice and the associated supervision activities are discussed, is a sign of how tentative and relatively under-developed the current work on enabling students to learn through practice still is. This situation exists not only in nursing but across the health care professions generally. The use of terms such as 'debriefing', 'critique', 'feedback' are not standardized, and as a rule there are no broadly agreed frameworks for considering and discussing student practice. This position was clearly illustrated in two cross-profession research projects (Fish, Twinn and Purr, 1990, 1991) and (Fish and Purr, 1991) where the findings demonstrated that no two professions used the same term for discussing practice.

The word 'debriefing' in this book is used to signify the activity of talking with the student or practitioner about practice that has been shared by both the supervisor and that person, and in which either was the main actor and the other the main observer. It is, of course, also possible for students to operate with their peers in respect of debriefing, and to develop self-assessment processes involving a debriefing approach which are discussed in detail in Chapter 7. Indeed, as Stengelhofen (1993) says: 'Peer feedback is important in laying down the concept that it is part of professional work to be observed and evaluated by one's own colleagues'.

'Debriefing', then, denotes a broad activity, and is preferable to terms like 'critique' ('crit') or 'feedback' because it is more neutral in tone, has more the sense of someone being helped to uncover and then work on what they know tacitly already, and fits more appropriately with the discussion that follows practice experience. Although the intention of feedback is to offer information to aid people in making adjustments to skills and the knowledge and emotional dimensions that affect them, the authors argue that it is nonetheless essentially judgemental. Ende (1983) (referred to in Stengelhofen, 1993, p. 154), suggests that 'feedback occurs when a student is offered insight into what he/she actually did', and compares this to a ballet-dancer learning in front of a mirror. Although this is a useful process, and ought to be part of any debriefing, it is not considered a separate category. Indeed we would suggest it will not necessarily further the student's learning if the insight is offered by the observer rather than emanating from the observed. The term 'critique', described below has been reserved for one subset of debriefing activities. It should be noted that video or audio recordings of the practice episode can be a very useful basis for debriefing.

Debriefing: procedures and issues

The process of debriefing

As with all scholarly matters, it is essential that debriefing should be carried out systematically and with discipline. Research carried out across a range of professions shows that this is rarely the case (Fish, Twinn and Purr, 1990, 1991; Fish and Purr, 1991). Since no agreed coherent view of debriefing is currently available in any health care profession, we offer, in the spirit of reflective practice, a *framework* (as opposed to a set model) for considering debriefing. This consists of a summary of the kinds of issues that need to be considered in debriefing. The supervisor's orientation to the technical–rational or professional artistry approach to professionalism will determine the character of the decisions made within each dimension.

A framework for considering debriefing

There are at least six dimensions to debriefing, as follows:

the aims	the orientation
the mode	the pedagogic style
the format	the nature and use of evidence

As McIntyre points out, debriefing (which he calls 'feedback') does different jobs at different stages in the student's development (McIntyre, 1994, p. 86). This means that each of these dimensions becomes more or less significant according to the supervisor's professional judgement in the specific situation.

Aims

The intentions of a debriefing after action are to help the student or practitioner to elicit meaning from the action. The purpose and focus for the *observation* will already have been decided when preparing for the observation, but the reasons for offering a debriefing can still vary. Some views about what supervision (and especially debriefing) consist of have been recorded by Watkins. Among them are the following:

- assisting someone to reflect critically
- guiding and supporting
- supporting and building
- leading by example (Watkins, 1992, p. 104).

Stengelhofen offers the following additional aims of supervision:

- to lead the student towards independent practice
- to build the student's confidence in his or her own skills
- to facilitate behavioural change
- to help the student arrive at a complete view of the professional role as well as to attend to the detail within it (Stengelhofen, 1993, p. 173).

But, as Lucas (1991) points out, in many supervisory situations there are likely to be conflicting aims for the supervisor and resulting tensions for the student or practitioner. He explores those problems which result from the supervisor's conflicting aims of being a resource for the reflective student/practitioner on the one hand and needing to offer the student/practitioner new insights unavailable through reflection on the other. Further, it is possible that while the supervisor is encouraging autonomous reflection, the result is that the student/practitioner merely goes through the motions of reflection in order to please the supervisor. There are also problems (in mode one supervision) of helping the student to learn at the same time as needing to assess him or her, and (in mode two), of facing additional conflicts of the supervisory relationship, particularly where the supervisor is the practitioner's line manager. The supervisor needs to be aware of these possibilities and to be flexible in responding to them during debriefing.

Orientation

It is also worth asking about whether the general orientation of the debriefing is to improve practice and/or foster professional judgement (refine action), or facilitate deliberation about issues or, if both, where the balance lies. Furthermore, the supervisor will need to consider whether debriefing focuses on the health needs of the patient or client identified by the student or practitioner, and the following practice intervention, or those health needs not identified by the supervisee, but apparent to the supervisor. This debate adds to the complexity of the debriefing process.

Modes

In discussing the approach to debriefing we would suggest that there are four main modes: a critique mode; a reflective mode; a formal assessment mode; and a self-assessment mode.

A critique mode offers 'a crit' of the episode of practice. Here the lead observer picks out salient points of positive and negative aspects of the observed practice and offers his or her own professional judgements about them and how the person observed might do better next time. In its best form 'critique' means, as it does of art critiques, an appreciation of the episode of practice. In its most instrumental form it might use a checklist of competencies, an activity sometimes referred to as 'feedback'.

A reflective mode offers both observer and observed a means of exploring what happened during practice and of thinking about how it might have been perceived, why it was as it was, the theories that underlay the actions and how to improve next time. Here the person observed has the opportunity to examine and refine his or her *own* professional judgements.

The formal assessment mode offers an official judgement of the episode of practice against a set standard. For students this standard will generally be determined by the learning outcomes identified for that practice area. Standards, as we have said, like competencies and outcomes, are notional and arbitrary however much they are presented as absolutes, and are central to the technical rational view of professionalism. The outcome of such assessment is formally recorded. This assessment may be formative (during the practice) or summative (at the end of the practice) – this latter is about passing or failing a student and acting as gatekeeper to the profession. This aspect will be dealt with in detail in Chapter 7.

The self-assessment mode offers a framework for the student, or indeed the practitioner, to take over the professional development role for him or herself.

Pedagogic style

Pedagogic style, broadly, is about the debriefer's supervisory style. This involves either *telling* the student/practitioner or *asking* him or her, and this in turn depends on whether the debriefer wants to demonstrate knowledge or lead the supervisee to discover it; and whether the debriefer wants to do all the work or facilitate that person's self-assessment.

Format

The format of the debrief can be oral or written. Students usually look for *both*, and Johns (1993) rightly in our view, argues that written notes of the debriefing process are essential in providing continuity to clinical supervision. However, in both oral and written feedback the order of questions or comments and the tone of them is vital. The format of the written record depends crucially on the intention of the observation and the preferred (or prescribed) pedagogic style. The written basis can be discursive/descriptive writing (longhand or note form), or filled-in forms. Forms are inevitably reductionist, but might enable the occasional focus on a small part of the episode of practice. Where a form has been filled in by the supervisor, its purpose, its role in the debriefing, and its significance after the debriefing need to be very clear. Some authors such as Haggar, Burn and McIntyre (1993) and Stengelhofen (1993) advocate forms as providing an objective basis for feedback. Research evidence suggests they are no less subjective than any other records (Twinn, 1989).

Nature and use of evidence

As indicated above (p. 116), there are two approaches during debriefing to the utilization of information collected during observation. On the one hand it is possible to offer it as *evidence* for critiques offered to the student or practitioner, on the other it is useful as the *basis for discussion* with that individual about a range of aspects of the practice. In the first case the information is treated as unproblematic 'hard' evidence about the student's or practitioner's success in performance. In the second it is seen as much less certain and as a means of exploring ideas and the roots of practice.

Interpersonal skills and debriefing

The role of counselling in supervision is one that remains open to debate. Some authors (e.g. Hawkins and Shohet, 1989; Stengelhofen, 1993; Swain, 1995) suggest that counselling should play a major role in supervision since the most difficult aspect of debriefing is talking to the student about issues that will not be comfortable for either party. Although in our view a greater priority is to develop an understanding of the deeper aspects of professional practice, certainly we do not dismiss the importance of such matters. This is particularly so since both experience and research evidence clearly demonstrate that debriefing must take account of the emotional dimension. Students, for example, often attend more to the tone of voice than to the content of debriefing and, in their role as assessors, some practitioners have difficulty in pointing out students' weaknesses and in failing them if it is necessary (Twinn, 1989). Stengelhofen refers to the useful work of Pickering (1987) in identifying ten behavioural skills that are associated with empathy, and which are of importance in debriefing. These are: attending/acknowledging; restating/ paraphrasing; reflecting; interpreting; summarizing, synthesis; supportive questioning; giving feedback; supporting; checking perceptions; being quiet (Stengelhofen, 1993, p. 161).

Again, of course, it is not the skills that are important but an understanding of the activities of supervision and the consequent professional judgement about when, how, and why to use them.

The following rules of thumb for the interpersonal aspects of debriefing are based upon but extended from the work of Rowie Shaw (see Shaw, 1992; Table 6.1).

Problems in debriefing

Although the significance of debriefing to the supervisory process has been acknowledged in nursing White and Ewan (1991), Watkins (1992) and Stengelhofen (1993) point out dangers and problems associated with debriefing. They make between them the following points and although these were made originally in relation to students they are equally pertinent when debriefing qualified practitioners.

- Students tend to remember the negative rather than the positive, and so good points need reinforcing.

Table 6.1 Some useful rules of thumb for debriefing

1 Always be clear about and be sure the student is clear about the intention of the observation.

2 Always try to make the observation and debriefing a learning situation for the student. Be positive as a first step. Never give negative feedback in public settings. If you offer negative feedback, show how things can be improved. Be specific, offer alternatives. (Suggest a new small target that will lead to success.)

3 Work *with* a student *not* on him or her. Avoid a power struggle. Don't take control over the interaction. We are all learners. Avoid suggesting that there are simple, right answers.

4 Don't tackle too many things at once – try to foster a sense of progress.

5 Get the comments and ideas from the student. Asking is usually better than telling.

6 Giving negative criticism or leading the student to focus on the things that did not work is sometimes important and should not be avoided. (It is tempting to avoid dealing with unsatisfactory work, but things will not improve without attention. There will come a time when it's too late to make your first negative comments.) Temper negative comments with praise and help student to see these as growing points. (Getting this balance right is a matter of professional judgement, wisdom and maturity.)

7 Use positive and warm non-verbal communication. Smile. Make eye contact. Don't be confrontational. *Listen* to the student.

8 Use evidence from the episode of practice in as objective a way as possible. Stick to facts presented in as neutral a way as possible. Use the evidence you have recorded (which may astonish the student) to provoke discussion.

9 Use open-ended questions, encourage frankness and share worries, uncertainties. Don't hide your reasons for questions or comments, or come at things too indirectly.

10 Always take account of as many dimensions of the episode of practice as possible (the intentions, the planning, the student's value-base, the student's experience, the different interpretation and perceptions of what has happened, the distinction between espoused theories and theories-in-use).

11 Your *own* different value-base and different skills are only of indirect importance. You are not trying to get the student to be more like you, but to be more fully him or herself (within professional parameters).

12 Don't be thrown by your own strong reaction to any individual part of the episode of practice. Don't let it colour the whole debriefing.

13 If you are asking the student to do something new or different as a result of the debriefing, be sure he or she understands what it is you are saying. Follow up by asking the student to say what he or she will aim at, and what first steps he or she will take.

14 If you are offering judgements about something, make their basis clear.

15 If the student counter-attacks you, don't rise. Try to see it from his or her point of view. Show that you will consider what is said. Explore it, clarify it. Illustrate your own position with simple facts and evidence from your

notes. Show that you are neutral at the personal level – or even that you are positive about the student as a person.

16 Set clear intentions (targets?) for the next supervisory session and even consider how the next observation will seek to help.

17 But the most difficult cases are those who are clearly not succeeding but not recognizing this. There comes a time when you must be firm.

- NB You must have provided them with very clear and unambiguous assessments and goals to retrieve the situation.
- There must be evidence that you have done so, that the student understands the situation and recognizes the deadlines.
- Keep careful notes of what you have said and what you have written and how you have sought to help, advise, counsel and offer sheltered learning opportunities.
- There may come a time when you have to use these as evidence that you have pointed out the same things again and again and that the student has failed to meet the goals you have set again and again.
- Then you can:
  describe the problem clearly to the failing student
  ask for the reasons for it
  listen sympathetically
  indicate *unambiguously* the failure
  offer help (tell them where to get it) in considering another career
  check that they have personal support from friends and family.
  After some anger they may well be secretly relieved.

- Students' views of what happened in the debriefing may be different from the supervisor's.
- This may be because students are not ready to accept the supervisor's critique.
- Supervisors can foist their presence and their views upon the student (which is unhelpful).
- Supervisors can offer apparently internally conflicting advice, or advice that conflicts with that of others in the practical setting, without giving time to look at these tensions and their reasons.
- Supervisors can demotivate students when they step in and take over something in practice or in discussion and then complain that the student has not contributed.
- Supervisors can provide too much supervisory presence.
- Supervisors can fail to give reasonable notice of practical or debriefing sessions.
- Supervisors can fail to warn students of problems until it is too late to put them right.
- Supervisors sometimes will not let the student have full control and responsibility.
- Supervisors can be resistant to student's new ideas (and not even explain why) (see Watkins, 1992; Stengelhofen, 1993).

Approaches to debriefing

Broadly there are two kinds of approach to debriefing, emanating from the two views of learning professional practice discussed above: the skills-based or competency-based approach, and reflective approaches emanating from the professional artistry view. The following examples are chosen to demonstrate each. They also, naturally, subscribe to very different views about the role of the supervisor. At a deeper level, moreover, they reveal very different attitudes to the role of the supervisor. These range from the view that the supervisor's major responsibility is to offer a model to the student and discuss what happened during practice at a rather superficial level, to the view that the supervisor is in a 'unique position in being able to provide precise feedback to individual students on all aspects of practical professional development' (Stengelhofen, 1993, p. 153). In addition, these views may also be influenced by whether the clinical supervision involves a student or qualified practitioner.

Two different approaches to debriefing are presented below: first an approach which is described as a model for structured reflection (Johns, 1993) and secondly the authors' own work called *Strands of Reflection* which is derived from cross-profession research, and which is already being used considerably in a range of health and paramedical professions.

Structured reflection

The approach to debriefing described by Johns (1993) as structured reflection attempts in his view to offer a framework for debriefing developed from the philosophy of reflective practice. However, the six stages offered as a guide in using the framework suggest a reductionist approach to the process of debriefing. This position is particularly emphasized in stage four of the framework in which a set list of rather narrow questions is provided for use by the supervisor or the supervisee, to facilitate reflection which is the focus of this stage of the framework. Although this approach may facilitate reflection at one level, in our opinion, it is very heavily supervisor-led and the prescriptive nature of the questions provides limited opportunity or guidance in developing debate of sufficient depth and breadth for students and practitioners to explore and understand the moral dimensions and the ambiguity, complexity and uncertainty of practice settings as described by Schön (1983). Indeed, it may lend itself to hijacking by managers as a tool in audit and appraisal and certainly is perceived by some practitioners as akin to these two processes (conference on reflective practice and patient outcomes, Macmillan, 1995). (Readers wishing to distinguish between reflective debriefing, and appraisal and audit, are referred to the framework on p. 128 above.)

In addition, the use of the term 'structured reflection', quite wrongly in our view, raises questions about the extent to which this approach readily fits with a philosophy of reflective practice and professional artistry. Indeed the use of the term 'structured' implicitly suggests the influence of a technical–rational approach to the development of the framework. Readers who wish to explore in more depth the approach proposed by Johns should refer to Johns (1993) and (1994).

In contrast to this approach to debriefing we offer below a framework that emphasizes reflection on action as a means of understanding better and thus improving practice, avoiding the reductionist approach of prescribed questions. First however we review other work on reflection.

In a previous publication by Fish (1989, pp. 76–80), a number of different approaches to reflection were highlighted. The most important of these include the work of Boud, Keogh and Walker, and William Pinar. The former offer a number of approaches to reflection and maintain that the goal of reconstructing experience is vital and that this will enable students to 'realise many things left undone, questions unasked and records incomplete' (Boud, Keogh and Walker, 1985, p. 10). Pinar (1986), also in the reconstructionist tradition, argues for the importance of autobiography. Other publications, including Carr and Kemmis (1986) and Pollard and Tann (1987), emphasize self-assessment, while Griffiths and Tann (1992), offer a series of five levels of reflection for investigating personal theory.

In occupational therapy there has been much important work on clinical reasoning (Mattingly and Fleming, 1994). For an overview of Mattingly and Fleming's four types of clinical reasoning (the procedural, the interactive, the conditional and the narrative) and of Schell and Cevero's three types (scientific, narrative and pragmatic reasoning) see Strong *et al.* (1995). Mattingly and Fleming developed their work because they felt that the education of OT students in America, with its emphasis on skills and procedures, did not accurately reflect the complexity and uniqueness of practice. McKay and Ryan (1995), on the basis of the three levels of reflection of Boud and Walker (1991), have developed guidelines for OTs for case stories which they say should be 'enhanced' during fieldwork visits to help students to think beyond the medical context to the personal. Ryan (1995) offers some useful types of questions (together with detailed examples) which can enhance learning during clinical placement. The main categories of question are: procedural, factual and precise; open-ended and broad; provocative and challenging; projective and conditional (Ryan, 1995, p. 251). She also draws on our work (detailed below) which she says 'can illuminate fieldwork experiences'.

The following (to which Ryan refers) draws from a research project which we directed in 1989–1991, and illustrates how a holistic approach to reflection might be supported by what is a *framework* of ideas.

Strands of reflection: one framework for debriefing

The following framework was developed as a result of a small project which looked in detail at student/tutor discussions of practice in health visiting and teaching (Fish, Twinn and Purr, 1990, 1991). It is based loosely on the early work of Zeichner and Liston (1987). There are four Strands (focuses) for thinking about action that has taken place, but they are complementary and only operate together. They are not intended to be used separately. They are Strands of one whole. They are: the factual; the retrospective; the sub-stratum; the connective strand. Together they can provide a holistic means of reflecting upon practice. They seek to aid broad interpretation of practice and the issues implicit in it rather than a narrow analysis of skills. The detail of each Strand is as follows.

A: The factual Strand

This is essentially descriptive and concerns itself with the student/practitioner providing a narrative of the events and processes of the practice situation (what happened, and what the student/practitioner felt, thought and did about it). These are, of course, recalled or reconstructed, but are thought through and presented as if the narrator is still within the situation. This Strand stresses the immediate and apparently piecemeal nature of the practice.

It should be noted that recapturing or reconstructing a complex situation chronologically in this way is not always easy, or straightforward. The mind/memory does not work like this. However, a disciplined attempt to relive/reconstruct it, preferably soon after the event, will usually enable the processes and events of the episode of practice to be ordered into a narrative. Such a process often enables the student/practitioner to recognize for the first time what actually has happened. If, after hearing the student's version, the supervisor offers his or her own, it establishes a genuinely shared basis from which further reflection can grow. (Many post-practice discussions that do not begin with this 'ground-clearing' run into difficulties later as points of disagreement about what actually happen begin to emerge.)

Broadly there are three kinds of detail involved: setting the scene; telling the story; and pin-pointing the critical incidents. The following offers some tentative ways of teasing out what is involved in this Strand.

1 *Setting the scene.* Briefly describe the context of the practice situation, referring to the intentions of the episode of practice and the practice setting.
2 *Telling the story.* Give a chronological reconstruction of the facts (the events and processes) of the practice situation as it happened (was experienced) step by step. (What happened, how did the student/practitioner think, feel and act, and why?)
3 *Pin-pointing the critical incidents.* This is about focusing upon and considering critically the key moments of the story. Identify and describe any incidents which particularly caused surprise, seemed to offer scope for learning, made the student/practitioner think twice. Say why the incident seemed 'critical'. Describe the resulting actions, thoughts, feelings.

B: The retrospective Strand

This is concerned with looking back over the entire events and processes of the practice as a whole and seeing patterns and possibly new meanings in them. It stresses deliberately the retrospective nature of the reflection, and draws theory from the practice. It develops sensitivity and imagination by asking how others such as professionals, patients or clients, and carers involved in the piece of practice might have viewed it and felt about it as a whole. It thus encourages the habit of considering a range of perspectives on the episode of practice as a whole. It is also, to some extent, evaluatory, in that the success of what happened as a whole should be considered. Again, after listening to the student's/practitioner's attempts to think in this way, the supervisor might offer further alternatives and stimulate further critical reflection about the issues raised, or introduce ideas that have not been considered by the student or practitioner.

The kinds of issues addressed within this Strand might include:

• What main patterns are visible in the piece of practice as a whole?
• What overall logic drove the piece of practice as a whole?
• What were the overall aims, intentions, goals and were they achieved?
• How might others (other professionals, patients, clients, carers) involved in the practice see it overall?
• What new knowledge was discovered/invented?
• What might an analysis of the language in the interaction tell one?
• What patterns were there of reason and/or motive?
• How did the learner-practitioner see him or herself as operating overall within the practice?

- What patterns were there of critical incidents, failures, successes, emotions, frustrations, limitations, constraints, coercions?

C: The sub-stratum Strand

This is concerned with discovering and exploring the assumptions, beliefs and value judgements that underlie the events and the ideas which emerge in Strands A and B above, and does not merely involve superficial criticism of what happened in practice. It seeks to broaden the considerations out beyond the technicalities of the events (the 'how' of the situation, i.e. the means), to a careful consideration of or deliberation about its intended goals (i.e. its ends). This widening out is assisted by consideration of a range of perspectives from formal theory and other professionals' personal experience and theory.

This strand encourages professionals to tolerate the idea that a range of views exists about procedures and that there is no right answer, and encourages them to face what lies beneath the surface of their practice. This is essential if the practitioner is to confront the crucial gaps to be found between beliefs and actions in their practice, and such confrontation is more likely to bring about real change than is any external decree. Here the supervisor might interact at each point with the student or practitioner, again offering further perspectives where possible.

Some of the following provide examples of the kind of questions which may be asked:

- What customs, traditions, rituals, beliefs, dogmas, prejudices were brought to/endemic in the situation? Where did they come from?
- What basic assumptions, beliefs, values lie under the actions and decisions reported in earlier strands?
- What beliefs are emerging about knowledge and how is it gained and used?
- What ideas about theory and practice are implicit in the practice and the reflections upon it?
- What moral and ethical decisions were embedded in the student's/practitioner's planning and in his or her actions in and reactions to the episode of practice?
- What beliefs and ideas lie under the kinds of evaluation and justification employed so far?
- What theories has the student/practitioner proceeded upon?

D: The connective Strand

This is concerned with how the practical and theoretical results of Strands A, B and C might be modified for use in future practice, or might or ought to relate to it, and with the practical implications of this. The information and understandings accrued via Strands A, B and C are now related to the wider world – that of other practical situations, the experiences, views, reflections, theorizings and actions of other professionals, other personal theory of the student or practitioner, and (via reading) that of formal theory. As a result of discussing these issues, the supervisor might press the student or practitioner to define a clear plan of action for the next episode of practice or contact with the patient or client.

The following are among relevant issues.

- What has been learnt from this situation as a whole, how has it related to past experiences, and how will it relate to future ones?
- How does this piece of practice relate to its historical, political and social contexts?
- How might both the thought and action specific to this practice situation be modified in the light of experience, further thought and further reading?
- How does this piece of practice relate to the traditions of practice in my profession?
- What tentative further theories might be developed for future action?
- What implications do these reflections have for future practice?

Ways of using Strands

It cannot be emphasized enough that these Strands offer only a framework for reflection. The questions suggested are an attempt to give the kind of flavour of the issues to be considered within each broad Strand. They are *not* a technical rational set of questions to be tackled in a routinized way. Equally the term 'Strands' is designed as a reminder that each is an element in an overall attempt to reflect upon practice and no one Strand is of use on its own.

In the authors' experience the framework needs practice by both supervisor and student or practitioner before it yields a full picture. The danger here is perhaps that the professional tackles only the first two (easier) Strands in the early stages. This would go against the spirit of the framework and, worse, would leave out vital issues of underlying values and beliefs. The sub-stratum Strand probes issues which are most often ignored in evaluation and appraisal, but it is the area in which our practice is most challenged.

This framework, then, is a means of facilitating learning through practice via debriefing. It is an attempt to give coherence and shape to the post-practice discussion which, as was found in the original project (Fish, Twinn and Purr, 1990), is often without shape and structure and is thus unsystematic. It is also a means of investigating practice and of pin-pointing aspects of practice that further need investigation.

In our view the framework has the potential to be useful to any professional practitioner who wishes to learn from a practice situation. It therefore is equally appropriate for a student, or a well-established professional. It might be of use in a simple piece of practice or for both student and supervisor in their own debriefing about their respective practices. It might be used by the student alone as a framework for

---

Task 6.1 Points for action associated with debriefing

These activities are designed to be tackled in chronological order.
1. Write a critique of your most recent debriefing of a student or a practitioner following an observation of practice. Use the following questions to help you:
   • What aspects of your observations did you share with the student/practitioner?
   • How many things have you highlighted for attention?
   • Did the student/practitioner manage to set new targets or aims?
   • What were the key differences between what you said to the student/practitioner and what you wrote for the student/practitioner? Why did they occur?
   • Did discussion with the student/practitioner teach you something new about the episode of practice? (Did it cause you to change your mind about any aspect of it?)
   • What did you expect would happen during the debriefing and after it? (Did it?)
   Encourage the student/practitioner to summarize your feedback session. Compare accounts.
2 Use 'Strands' on an episode of your own practice, paying particular attention to Strands C and D; either talk it through with a colleague, or write about it.
3 Watch an episode of practice carried out by a student or practitioner (or video a student/practitioner and sit with some colleagues to watch it). First, pinpoint some issues about the practice to which you would wish to alert the student. Then, using 'Strands', select the key questions and/or devise your own based on 'Strands', that would be most helpful in getting the person observed to see for him or herself the important points you have highlighted. List these questions in the order you would use them with the student. (Where possible compare your ideas with a colleague's.)
4 Watch a student/practitioner carry out an episode of practice, making your own diary notes of key events. Then, using 'Strands', explore with the student both the practice and the Strands framework. (Perhaps then ask the questions suggested in the first task above.)

thinking or writing a journal/diary. It is often best used to start with in partnership with someone else who is also seeking to investigate their practice. It might also be used as an alternative way of investigating a piece of practice that has already been highlighted by some other means (such as self-appraisal). Readers are now directed to Task 6.1.

Further reading

Boud, D., Keogh, R. and Walker, D. (1985). *Reflection: Turning Experience into Learning*. Kogan Page.

Griffiths, M. and Tann, S. (1992). Using reflective practice to link personal and public theories. *Journal of Education for Teaching*, **18**, 69–84.

Johns, C. (1993). Professional supervision. *Journal of Clinical Management*, **1**, 9–18.

Johns, C. (1994). Guided Reflection. In *Reflective Practice in Nursing* (A. Palmer, S. Burns and C. Bulman, eds) pp. 116–130, Blackwell Scientific Publications.

Pinar, W. (1986). 'Whole, bright, deep with understanding.' Issues in qualitative research and autobiographical method. In *Recent Developments in Curriculum Studies* (P. H. Taylor, ed.) pp. 3–18, NFER/Nelson.

White, R. and Ewan, C. (1991). *Clinical Teaching in Nursing*. Chapman and Hall.

7
Considering competencies and assessing professional competence in practice

Introduction

The assessment of professional competence in clinical settings in health care professions is a complex and problematic matter. It is further complicated by whether the supervisor operates in Mode 1 with either students newly preparing to enter the profession or with qualified practitioners who are completing a post-registration programme (such as that of the specialist practitioner described by the English National Board for Nursing, Midwifery and Health Visiting (ENB, 1995)), or whether the supervisor operates in Mode 2, working with a colleague in a shared professional setting as a means of professional development associated with being in post.

In both Mode 1 situations, the supervisor has the responsibility of deciding whether the student has achieved the learning outcomes determined by the professional body (the UKCC, CSP, COT, or the British Acupuncture Accreditation Board (BAAB) on behalf of the (BAcC), for example) and therefore can be admitted to the appropriate professional register. Naturally, the responsibility of the supervisor in fulfilling a gatekeeping role is more complex with the qualified practitioner. This is discussed in detail in Chapter 8. In both cases, however, the supervisor is required to assess the student or practitioner formally by means of assessment tools set down in the relevant course.

In respect of the supervisor operating in Mode 2, there are three recent moves which highlight the increasingly significant role of the supervisor in assessing the continuing competence of the practitioner, and/or indicate the potential for the development of this across professions. These are:

- the requirement of recent legislation that all nurse practitioners maintain a personal profile as part of their continuing registration (UKCC, 1995b)
- the emphasis in government documents on nursing of the importance of clinical supervision

- the beginnings of the use of profiling for professional development purposes in other health care professions.

The central focus of this chapter is therefore on practical assessment. Section two suggests some principles of procedure for assessing students against competencies or the learning outcomes determined by the various key bodies associated with individual health care professions. Section three looks at providing a more balanced assessment of the student to supplement competency-based assessment, and proposes a holistic approach to the assessment of reflective practice. Section four focuses briefly on the supervisor as assessor. First however, in section one, as a prior concern, the problematic nature of assessment itself is probed and some principles related to assessment are set out.

Assessment: complexities and problems

The problematic nature of assessment

Although assessment is frequently portrayed by a range of different bodies as a simple matter, like all aspects of education, it is in fact complex and problematic. (See Edwards and Knight (1995) for a full discussion of the flawed nature of the assessment of competencies in the context of higher education and the case for increased collaboration between higher education providers and professional groups committed to student learning.) In order to familiarize readers with the nature of assessment and some of the conflicting principles that lie under the surface, this section will begin with a review of two contrasting approaches to assessment, and move from there to consider the assessment of students and then the assessment of qualified practitioners, and in passing will comment upon the relationship between these three.

Contrasting approaches to assessment

The following two contrasting approaches to the process of assessment attempt to demonstrate some of its conflicting concerns.

In an extreme version of what might be described as the training or delivery model of learning, such as that experienced with some of the programmes offered by the National Council for Vocational Qualification (NCVQ), the trainer is responsible for 'delivering' the learning and assessing whether or how well it has been received by the learner. (Here it should be noted that in spite of the somewhat ironic use of the term 'vocational' in the title, the jobs for which this qualification was originally designed fell well short of anything that might have been called professions.) Indeed, Langford (1995), arguing for the use of NVQ as a basis for complementary medicine programmes, talks not about 'professions' but about 'occupations'. Jones and Moore (1993) see the competency movement in the context of change in the social control of expertise in society, and view the move by the National Council for Vocational Qualifications into graduate level occupations (NVQ level 5) as a method of translating expertise into competencies and thus controlling professional practice.

In this version of training, then, assessment is most often summative, offering a summary of the learning achieved at the end of course, and formal, being a self-contained unit in an artificial or unfamiliar situation which happens outside, or after, the learning itself. It is 'applied' by the trainer to the learner. It is either norm-referenced (where the learner is compared against the standard of the group (or nation), or criterion-referenced (where the learner is required to meet criteria already set down about what should be learnt). The purpose of such assessment is to assess (measure) the learner against a standard, and for the trainer to check-up on the learner – usually on the learner's recall or skills acquisition, and to classify his or her performance on the basis of the assessment.

These all-pervasive 'standards', currently considered so important by many professional groups, are created on the basis of the norm for the group or are devised on the basis of competencies. However, they are merely external reference points which at bottom are notional. In student assessment they rely on the notion of an average performance of a group (the group size ultimately being arbitrary) in norm-referenced assessment, and in criterion-referenced assessment they are devised on the basis of 'those aspects of performance which can be assessed . . . or the learning programme which result in an efficient performance' (see Mansfield, 1989, p. 30). This so-called 'task model' of standards provides a description of what the individual would have to do in order to demonstrate competence, but is in fact inadequate for all but the most basic of tasks (see Mitchell, 1989).

Such learning is not only in danger of being short term, but is also not owned by, and barely touches or stays with the learner – many readers may have experienced examinations of this sort. Indeed such assessment involves the supervisor (or examiner) evaluating a 'performance' which is visible and quantifiable, instead of focusing on long-term and in-depth understanding, which although it might be preferable, is less visible and is notoriously difficult to make evident as the basis of formal assessments. Equally unattended to in this approach to assessment is the holistic view of the learner as a human being with personality and emotions, interests and difficulties, strengths and weaknesses. As

Shifrin says, while writing about setting standards for acupuncture via the BAAB, there is 'a danger of depending too much on measurement of competencies without a counterbalancing view of the inner qualities of the practitioner' (Shifrin, 1993, p. 15). There is no interest here in enabling learners to come to grips with self-knowledge, neither is there real concern to enable the learner to engage in self-assessment. The purpose of this approach to assessment in the authors' view is to divide up and label learners for bureaucratic and political rather than educational ends.

By stark contrast, but equally problematic, is the model of learning and assessment that places emphasis entirely on the processes of learning at the expense of visible outcomes, and where assessment is formative (simply as an ongoing tool to support learning), informal, and part of the day-to-day educational activity of the practice setting. This approach fits uncomfortably with the current national obsessions for empirical evidence, public standards and the comfort of what seems to be certain knowledge, and is of no use where categorizing learners is thought necessary. It values the long-term nature of education and acknowledges the individual needs of the learner, and the subjectivity of evaluation, to the point where no tangible evidence is recorded formally, where assessment is merely continuous informal feedback to the learner and where the emphasis is on the holistic individual. No interest is taken in progress against national standards but only against the learner's previous attainments (assessment is self-referenced, or 'ipsative', and recorded – often by the learner – in individual, learner-centred profiles). There are many arguments against this approach, including the doubtfulness of being able to capture on paper 'the whole person' (see Law, 1984; Broadfoot, 1986; Hitchcock, 1989).

Both of these two extremes, then, represent diverging and even conflicting trends in assessment and very different ways of valuing human beings. The one emphasizes psychometric tests and the evaluation, labelling and categorizing of individuals against a standard, the other attempts to nurture achievements and understanding, and capture and celebrate the wide range of personality of the learner. One focuses on specific behaviours as achievements, the other values the multifaceted account of a complex individual. One records specific learning that has happened, the other sees assessment as a tool of educational development, ultimately providing for an autonomous self-knowing, self-assessing learner.

Having presented the foregoing contrasts, we are now in a position to offer the following statements about and principles of assessment.

First then, it can be said that assessment is a very powerful set of tools. When used as part of a course, the purposes for assessment should relate to the purposes of the teaching and learning and the processes of assessment should be designed as an integral part of the course. Assessment can be used for a variety of ends and it behoves practitioners involved in professional education to be aware of the moral as well as the educational dimensions of these uses. Thus it can be argued that assessments in which methods and timing are inappropriate to the nature of what is being learnt and to the needs of the supervisor and the learners, can seriously distort both what is to be learnt and what has been achieved in learning.

From this it is possible to argue for the following set of principles (which has been influenced by the work of Bridges, Elliott and Klass, 1986), and which might be applied to all learners in any educational practice setting.

1 The purposes of assessment should be carefully considered. As well as enabling classification and categorization of learners, it might be a useful tool *during* learning, assisting learners in gaining self-knowledge and self-assessment, assisting supervisors in adjusting subsequent supervision, and helping learners to recognize the achievements they have secured.
2 Thus, any assessment procedures employed ought to assist – even maximize – the professional development of the learner, whatever other intentions they also fulfil.
3 Since a limited focus on performance in learning might distort what is recorded about learner achievement, the use of multiple perspectives on learning events and situations and the use of a variety of assessment tools might be valuable.
4 Holistic judgements about learners, inferred from a wide range of evidence, is likely to be more useful in assisting later supervision and learning than the narrow judgements based only on measurable performance.
5 Checking assessment judgements against other knowledge, including the learner's self-assessment, might increase the accuracy of that assessment.

These principles, although very general and developed from educational literature, are highly relevant to the assessment of student practitioners in health care professions. In addition, assessment processes in such professions must also take account of the nature of professional knowledge generally and of the specific nature of such knowledge in each profession, as well as of the necessary preparation and procedures which allow entry to a profession. They need to provide evidence, for example, of whether student practitioners can *exercise* their practical knowledge (whether they can successfully employ critical analysis, clinical reasoning, professional judgement, and whether they can solve unique professional problems, *in situ*). Students on preregistration courses must also be able to be assessed summatively and if necessary excluded from the profession.

Assessment in professional practice must fulfil a gatekeeping purpose. For example, in nursing, assessment achieves this gatekeeping role by requiring student practitioners to meet the learning outcomes determined by the UKCC. In physiotherapy and occupational therapy, as well as in preparation for alternative medicine professions, there are similar mechanisms. The achievement of these outcomes in both theory and practice allows the student practitioner to be admitted to the appropriate professional register. The development of learning outcomes as a method of assessment for entry to some professions could be argued as a progressive move from the previously held competencies required for professional registration. However, it can also be argued that in reality there is little difference between the achievement of learning outcomes or competencies since in both cases representatives of the profession have determined in considerable detail what *they* consider constitutes good practice and a safe practitioner, and this (almost inevitably) ignores the context specific aspects of good practice and the invisible processes of professional judgement. In fact it is possible to argue that 'criteria', 'competencies' and 'learning outcomes' are three terms for the same thing.

Indeed, when drawing up learning outcomes or competencies as the criteria for beginning practitioners, skills are predominantly portrayed as the major concern. This assumes a commonly agreed version of good practice, implies that assessing the performance of skills is a simple, objective matter, and erroneously suggests that skills are both unrelated to context and at the same time generic and generalizable to all contexts. In fact, as McIntyre points out in his discussion of the criterion-referenced assessment of teaching, the kind of assessment designed for student teachers crucially depends on how the activity of teaching is seen (McIntyre, 1989, pp. 65–6). For example, is it understood best as a set of personal characteristics, is it a skilled craft, a theory-based technology or a political activity? He reminds us too that there is no agreed *theory* of competencies, nor even a list of generally agreed principles, on the basis of which to derive a list of requirements. Benner (1984) provides a similar argument in her discussion of the definition of competence and the competencies required of the expert practitioner in nursing, though she offers in their place a putative series of levels of practice, which itself does not stand up to critical scrutiny as breaking away from the technical–rational view of professionalism.

To focus on the performance of skills as the practical basis for entry to a profession is a seductive idea. The apparent advantages are that they lend themselves to clear statements about what learners should know, be able to do or to demonstrate, how and against what criteria they are assessed, and provide simple reporting to students, other supervisors, colleagues and employers. They are also claimed to open up more flexible ways of learning via units and modules, although this is arguable. Further, using competencies for assessment appears to improve basic skills in the short term (though at the expense of the long term); it is easily organized into a bureaucratic model for administrative purposes, thus apparently increasing efficiency; it appears to lead to objective assessment (but in fact hides value judgements); and is about improving the performance of basic skills (though at the expense of understanding the complexities of when and how to use them). Garland defends them stoutly. He argues that they 'ensure the maintenance of objective, reified standards' and that they *can* enable wider issues and processes to be used and can be a basis from which learner-centred approaches and learner autonomy can be developed (Garland, 1994, pp. 17–18). He also (correctly) maintains that criteria of this sort are being adopted for most vocational qualifications in the further education sector and in higher education they are now well under way in the shape of General National Vocational Qualifications (GNVQs). He argues for *processes* to be enshrined as competencies, 'to ensure that . . . personal and professional developments are identified as crucial' (Garland, 1994, p. 19). He seems unaware, however, of the philosophical distinction between competence and competencies (see above, p. 48).

The real problems, however, are that competencies entirely 'fail to account for much of what teachers [and all professionals] do and more importantly, why they do it' (see Chown and Last, 1993, p. 15), and lead to 'serious difficulties in training and education' (see Ashworth and Saxton, 1990, p. 3). In nursing, occupational therapy and acupuncture, learning outcomes (or competencies) may be broadly focused in what they set out to assess, but they also ignore the importance of the nature of professional activity and professional knowledge, the importance and complexities of educational understanding, the nature of the practitioner as a person, the importance of personality to success in practice and the activities of theorizing, reflecting and learning during action. The competency-based approach also fails to identify whether the student is learning and refining practice as opposed to going through trained motions. In addition, it shows no interest in the investigation of practice as a basis for improving practice. It is unable to recognize the essentially incomplete, uncertain, and collaborative nature of professional activity, ignores professional judgement and risk-taking, and takes no account of the moral dimensions of practice because it does not pursue reasons, motives, theories, values. Further, it takes no account of beginning practitioners' own theories.

Assessing the student and qualified practitioner

In addition, then, to the competencies that are required to be assessed (and which in themselves are a very basic – necessary but not sufficient – requirement), it is vital that students are assessed in ways which respond to these matters and which take account of other principles of assessment and the practicalities of operating assessment. These same issues also hold for the assessment of the performance of qualified practitioners.

The assessment of performance among qualified practitioners is more complex, since although the principles underpinning the assessment process are equally relevant, the processes of clinical supervision that should be adopted with this group of practitioners remain uncertain. Indeed, although the need for clinical supervision of qualified practitioners has become accepted, doubts remain about its role and function. As a result there are still tensions about the purposes of it (for professional development or for covert managerial control); about who shall be the supervisor; about the bases for supervision; about who owns the information; and about who shall be made privy to it. It is interesting that these issues have also been faced in other professional

---

Task 7.1 Points for action and reflection

1 Choose an episode of practice you have recently carried out and list briefly, perhaps against a time entry, your own *activities* during that episode and then add, in another colour, your thoughts, worries, questions, puzzles, feelings, processes of decision-making or clinical reasoning.

2 Would you have done or said anything differently if there had been either a mode 1 or mode 2 supervisor observing and recording your practice?

3 How might a mode 1 or mode 2 supervisor, using a checklist of basic skills to be ticked, have recorded your work? What might have been missing from this record?

4 Would there be differences in your response to questions 2 and 3, according to the two different modes of supervision?

5 Were there any events in that episode of practice that someone observing but not discussing that practice afterwards might have misunderstood/misinterpreted?

6 If your 'practitioner effectiveness' were to be generalized from that one episode of practice, what would be said of you? How far is this a fair general picture?

7 If three sample episodes of practice were observed, chosen at random from your work, would the generalizations from them about your practitioner effectiveness be any fairer?

groups such as teaching and academics in higher education, where appraisal has become a requirement for staff (Task 7.1).

In the discussion above we have argued that assessment of student practitioners and qualified practitioners is not sensibly nor usefully attended to by means only of learning outcomes or competencies. However, they currently provide a fundamental basis for assessing professional practice and therefore must be used during the assessment process. The following discussion describes how this may be achieved, before looking at wider approaches.

Using competencies as part of assessment

Recent developments in nurse education and the preparation of OTs have shown an attempt to move away from the previous competency-based approach to assessment, but the extent to which learning outcomes differ fundamentally from competencies remains open to question. In addition, the development of NCVQ, which is also based upon competencies derived from task analysis, and its rapid extension into professional contexts and higher education, reveals the strength of the current influence of competencies. The following discussion therefore identifies some practical issues and indicates some possible principles of procedure for clinical supervisors most of whom have to use competencies at the moment as an approach to assessing students' performance in practice.

Using competencies: some practical issues

It will be remembered that competence (in the singular) relates to the holistic approach to professional capacity which cannot be reduced to individual competencies, while a competency-based approach to education assumes that practice can be atomized into individual skills (see above, p. 48). Once again to clarify some of these ideas it is useful to turn to the teaching profession where Hartley (1992) usefully summarizes the assumptions and character of competency-based teacher education.

In competency-based ITE, the teacher is seen as the significant agent in causing intellectual development in the learner and it is the teacher's actions and transactions with learners that affect the rate and quality of learning. Competencies therefore emphasize the role of the teacher and expect the observer to focus on this. Competencies assume that the role of the teacher can be described in terms of specific, observable acts or behaviours, and that these can be learnt and put into operation by intending teachers. Assessment is thus based upon performance of pre-specified and agreed competencies, seen in the 'field' setting. The focus of observation needs to be shared with the student in advance and levels of mastery of the behaviours are expected to be measured against a clear scale. Students should be instructed in these behaviours in advance of assessment and should be very clear about all the criteria used in assessment. Assessment should be based on performance, though knowledge 'may be taken into account'. Benner in an early publication on competency-based testing in nurse education, while acknowledging the limitations of this approach, highlights the fact that competencies can be drawn from actual nursing performance rather than expert opinion (Benner, 1982).

Some of the practical issues associated with competency-based assessment are as follows.

1 It is not clear how the competencies relate together, nor whether stronger aspects of one may be allowed to compensate weaker aspects of another. (This is not a problem in more holistic assessment.)

2 Likewise there is no clear ranking of competencies.

3 It is not clear what counts as evidence for 'passing' a competency. How often, for example, must a skill be seen, by how many different assessors, and in how many variable contexts, before it can be deemed 'mastered'?

4 How should a student be assessed who can score as passable on all of the competencies individually, but who is unable to establish a therapeutic relationship with patients or clients or who fails to develop a rapport with them?

5 How does the assessor record the problems of a student who will learn to go through the motions of the required (known about and trained for) competencies, but who does not really subscribe to them or clearly does not intend to use them once he or she has passed?

6 Competencies (abilities) 'are not attributes of individuals which exist independently of the contexts in which they are realised. They are qualities of the relationship between the individual and the context in which she or he operates', and the achievements they signify 'depend upon the individual (a) understanding the context as an opportunity to exercise a certain ability and (b) understanding himself or herself as capable of realising that ability' (see Bridges, Elliott and Klass, 1986, p. 230).

7 Competencies can only be fairly assessed by studying performance in a *variety* of contexts, and then generalizations about them should be 'the outcome of a comparative study of performance-in-context and not of a process of abstraction from context' (Bridges, Elliott and Klass, 1986, p. 230).

8 Assessment of performance should take account of the individual's personal interpretation of the context of his or her performance. It

would be invalid to label a student incapable of a skill because of its absence if the student had 'read' the situation as not requiring it.

9 High quality performances are those which utilize those personal capacities and which call forth abilities which are appropriate to and crucial for success in the given context, not ones which satisfy a pre-specified checklist of attributes of a good practitioner.

Some suggested principles of procedure

The following principles of procedure are suggested as a guide for those who have to operate competencies.

1 Competencies might be regarded as a basic requirement, in two senses – as a base-level for assessing students and as one part of assessment.
2 This part of the assessment might be accepted as only attending to a very limited range of issues, which may be supplemented in a number of ways. ('Other ways' might consist of tapping understanding, of probing the moral concerns and of checking whether the interpretation of the 'facts' is accurate.) The third section of this chapter offers some help with this.
3 Careful consideration should be given to what is understood by the criteria required by the professional statutory bodies and any levels of criteria, measurements and other operational features suggested within the course. These ought to be agreed and understood in common across supervisors and students from the beginning of their professional relationship.
4 The assessment operated should clearly assess what it sets out to assess, and not something quite different. For example, to 'train' students in a skill or competency and then assess an episode of practice in which the major focus is on the use of that particular skill, might be to assess the student's ability to please the assessor and the assessor's ability to train the student. But it is unlikely to assess the ability to draw upon the skill intelligently in an unexpected but appropriate moment.
5 The purpose for assessment should be understood by all parties on each occasion. Such purposes might include the deliberate attempt by the supervisor to check on abilities already well-observed informally, or to check on the absence of earlier problems originally made in non-assessment contexts.
6 The assessment should, wherever possible, be a learning experience. Equally, it should be clear to the student in which situations competencies are being assessed and when he or she is free to experiment and take risks.

7 It is important to be systematic about observation and have a clear idea of how broad a range of situations you will be seeking to observe the student in, what range of observation tools and data you will be drawing on and how many assessors should see him or her.

8 Systematic ways should be found of taking account of and recording clearly as part of the assessment the *context* in which the student was working.

9 Simple negative inferences should never be drawn from negative situations. For example an individual's apparent failure to respond appropriately in a given context might stem from a different view of what was necessary, or from self-doubt rather than actual lack of the competencies. An important part of the data of performance assessment includes checking interpretations of context and under-standings about self on the part of the student.

10 The list of competencies can be used both formatively and summa-tively (during an episode of practice and at the end of it). It is worth starting, however, *not* with the words on the page, but with the qualities and abilities of the student, and then filling in the list from these. In other words, the use of the list in a practical setting as an assessment tool is very limited, but it can be used as part of the reporting activity, or as an agenda for discussion and negotiation.

11 What counts as evidence of competencies needs to be carefully considered and what it is really evidence of needs to be clarified. (Avoid generalizing from a single context. Success in one context may both look and be quite different from success in another. Some contexts are much easier to look good in than others, and the simple 'average' grade gained from seeing a range of contexts may not be a fair indication of the quality of the student.)

12 Achievements should be seen and reported as outcomes of the inter-action between the context and the student.

13 Simply completing the list as numbers or ticks is virtually useless. The list can be used as a guide but comments need to be added. The notion of levels and measurements should be resisted if possible. Assessment on a pass/fail basis is less prone to disagreement. Especially seek to avoid putting everything as 'average and there-fore 3' on a 1 to 5 scale, which is often demanded in an attempt to 'profile competency'. This means producing a simple and highly reductionist document based solely on the given competencies. A much more balanced form of profiling, where instead of starting with ideas about practice, the process of profiling begins with the human involved, is discussed in the section below.

It now remains to turn to the wider approach to assessment and to look at how reflective practice might be assessed.

Assessing professional competence

In order to assess something it is important to understand its nature. On the basis of all that has been said so far, we would wish to argue for a holistic view of the nature of professional competence, and a recognition of a wider role for the practitioner than that of a mere 'safe deliverer' of care, which is what lies at the heart of a competency-based approach to assessment. (The word 'competence' is being used here in David Carr's sense, see above page 49).

We suggest that good – or quality – work in professional practice encompasses not the pre-specified list of individual competencies that take no account of context, but a *repertoire* of skills, abilities, capacities, professional knowledge, personal attributes, personality and ability to work with other professionals, together with what determines their appropriate employment according to the context in which the professional is employed (namely flexibility, educational understanding, moral awareness and professional judgement). Further, the model of professionalism which espouses reflective practice, to which we subscribe, contributes some additional dimensions to the character of professional practice. It emphasizes reflection (including ability to theorize during practice) and professional artistry (the wisdom to 'read', the flexibility to react to, and the ability to improvise in response to, the demands of the specific context). It also values the ability, via reflection-in- and on-action, to refine practice, and the associated knowledge and ability to investigate practice. Indeed, Winter argues that 'professional workers in human affairs can only practise effectively and justly if they *learn* from the individual cases in which they are involved, since their expertise, as a body of knowledge, is always inadequate and incomplete with respect to its objects and purposes' (Winter, 1989, p. 192). Assessment thus ought to take account of this too.

Finally, we would argue that contrary to many current views, these aspects of professionalism are not a 'second level' of activity for the practitioner to learn after he or she has 'mastered the basic skills', but are an integral part of what is to be learnt from the beginning of a course. As Russell argues, good work in professionalism *always* involves more than basic *skills* (see Russell, 1989). Thus, moral concerns and understanding of the values, beliefs and assumptions that underlie actions, are not attributes that a practitioner can add on to practice at a later stage in professional development. They are part of the very person one is, and there is a moral imperative that they should be attended to from the very beginning of professional preparation.

What we propose then is assessment which seeks evidence that student practitioners have the ability and potential to operate as competent professionals, and are able to ensure that patients and clients in a range of varied contexts receive high quality care appropriate to their health needs. Such assessment should also respond to student practitioners as complex and different individuals rather than demanding the same from all. This approach to assessment is therefore not concerned with the strengths and weaknesses of students' *individual* skills (except where one such clearly affects the overall competence, or where a detailed analysis is needed in order to isolate and practise a skill for some reason).

An example of the *practical* differences in focus between this approach to assessment and the competency-based approach is captured in Table 7.1, devised originally to enable students to consider their own practice from different perspectives and to improve their self-assessment procedures. Here, the right hand side offers examples of the kinds of objectives-focused, competency-based, standard (rather closed) questions to be asked about an episode of practice (to ensure that it reaches a basic level of acceptability), the left hand side suggests the sorts of questions that a reflective practitioner might ask to probe the quality of practice – given the purpose of both the episode of practice and the assessment of it. The two sides *do not relate to each other directly*, but are presented together to facilitate comparison. Although the questions are posed in a self-assessment form, they could also be used by an observer during practice. The contrasting texture of their language is interesting (see Table 7.1 on p. 156).

Given all these issues, how then might reflective practice be assessed?

A holistic approach to assessing reflective practice

First, we wish to suggest that the purpose of assessment in all professional practice should be to aid the educational development of the student as well as to fulfil the gatekeeping requirement, and that thus assessment should always be concerned with raising quality in practice rather than with a basic level of acceptability. Secondly, influenced by the work of Shulman (1987), but going beyond his seven types of professional knowledge, we suggest nine aspects of professionalism to act as focuses for assessment (i.e. aspects that the supervisor might actively seek). We also suggest four modes of assessment which describe the activities engaged in by the students and the supervisor as a means to assessment and which offer a range of possible processes of assessment for both supervisor and student to operate. In addition, we propose a different style of assessment from the quantification associated with measuring competencies.

Throughout the students' educational experience, the main purpose for assessment should be kept in mind, the individual student and the context should be taken account of, and the overall pattern of success

Table 7.1 Two approaches to assessment

Active reflective practice (takes account of purposes and context)	*Evaluating competencies* (in context of statutory learning outcomes)
What does my planning tell me about my values / beliefs / theories / moral stances and my expectations of the context?	Have I identified social and health implications of events such as pregnancy, disease, disability, for individuals and communities?
Why am I focusing on this piece of practice?	Have I recognized factors contributing to the social, physical and mental well being of patients and clients?
What actually happened? (several versions possible) What critical incidents can I pin-point? What do they tell me?	Have I made use of literature/research to inform practice?
How did I respond to client's queries/ comments? What does this tell me?	Have I appreciated the influence of social, political and cultural factors? Have I understood the requirements of legislation for the practice of nursing?
Are there any significant patterns in what happened?	Have I used appropriate communication skills to allow caring relationships?
What theories, values, beliefs lay under my practice?	Have I initiated and conducted therapeutic relationships with patients/clients?
What role did improvisation play?	
What role did professional judgement play? What key decisions did I make during practice?	Have I identified health related learning needs of patients/clients?
What were their practical and moral bases?	Have I participated in health promotion? Have I understood the ethics of health care? Have I understood the responsibilities ethics impose on nursing practice?
What theories and practices from other people will enlighten my understanding of this?	Have I identified the needs of patients/ clients to enable them to progress from dependence to maximum independence or a peaceful death?
How can I systematically investigate this practice further?	Have I identified the physical, spiritual, psychological and social needs of patients and clients?
Are there any prescriptions about practice that I should take account of?	Have I devised, implemented and evaluated a plan of individualized care?
How does what happened link to previous and future practice?	Have I demonstrated the application of the principles of a problem-solving approach to practice?
What broader issues does this all raise for membership of a profession?	Have I functioned effectively as a team member?
How do the professional development issues relate to those associated with management responsibilities?	Have I referred matters not within my sphere of competence? Have I assigned appropriate duties to others? Have I supervised, taught and monitored assigned duties?

(How will this affect the next plans?)

(or failure) in caring for patients and clients should be seen as mattering most of all. The notion of 'repertoire' which is used here denotes the overall pattern of characteristics or skills which together make for overall success. No absolute order of priority is suggested.

The focuses for assessment

The nine aspects of professionalism derive directly from the nature of professionalism suggested above. The sort of evidence that the supervisor might seek about students consists of patterns of behaviour across a range of practice activities as well as practice contexts, at a level appropriate to a beginning practitioner (or less if the student is not near the end of the course).

The aspects are:

1 The student's personal repertoire (personal characteristics; personality; general knowledge-base; self-knowledge and ability to improve it – this to include: self-awareness, sensitivity to others and ability to engage in balanced self-assessment). (McLaughlin, quoting Hare (1993), lists: distance, humility, courage, impartiality, open mindedness, empathy, enthusiasm, imagination, and disinterestedness (see McLaughlin, 1994, p. 159.)

2 The student's subject knowledge-base drawn from those disciplines needed as part of professional activities and the implications of such knowledge for patient/client care.

3 The student's skills/competencies repertoire (as required by the statutory bodies).

4 The student's professional knowledge (of professionally related theory, frameworks for practice, practice contexts and practice outcomes).

5 The student's professional understanding (knowledge to enable the selection of appropriate practice strategies, ethical dimensions of practice, moral awareness and ability to recognize the moral stance beneath decisions and actions).

6 The student's professional judgement (flexibility and decision-making (clinical reasoning) about when and how best to employ the personal and skills repertoire to provide appropriate patient and client care in a given context).

7 The student's professional artistry (the wisdom to 'read' a situation, the ability to respond to it, and the capacity to improvise).

8 The student's capacity for professional collegiality (ability to work with a wide range of fellow professionals).

9 The student's capacity for professional development (ability to theorize in practice and to recognize theories underlying own

actions; awareness of own espoused theories and theories-in-use; ability to reflect on own practice; ability to learn through practice; ability to investigate own practice; ability to operate practitioner enquiry activities at a simple level within own practice setting; ability to improve and refine practice and to recognize and work on mistakes).

Arguably, the supervisor is seeking, long term, to hand over assessment to the student and it is therefore appropriate that the capacity for self-knowledge and the ability to engage in self-assessment are both fostered and monitored as a part of almost all the assessment procedures adopted. Ways of enabling the student to gain self-knowledge (to know what he or she stands for, to clarify principles, ideals, to review personal attributes, to come to terms with uncertainties as well as certainties), ought to permeate all practical and dialectical aspects of the student's course. Opportunities for engaging in self-assessment of practice should be built into all planning of patient and client care, should be central to reflective practice and should also be fostered by a range of the modes of assessment discussed below. These modes, used together, will offer supervisors useful evidence of the student's self-knowledge and capacity for self-assessment.

Modes of assessment

There is a range of activities in which the supervisor and student can engage in order to highlight these aspects of the student's professionalism. They are: observation by the supervisor of the student's practice; a range of kinds of discussion of practice observed; a range of student writing; and practical investigations of practice and/or learning by the student.

Observation by the supervisor under this holistic approach is a different activity from that in competency-based assessment. Here, the supervisor is not present in the practice setting to measure, count, and record performance in 'objective' terms 'for the record's sake', but as one who either shares the experience of the episode of practice, or seeks to collect information about an aspect of it (for, and at the student's request), in order to seek to make sense of it and to see how to help the student to make sense of it afterwards. As Garland states in the context of teacher education, 'agreement needs to be reached between tutors and student-teachers' about what evidence is needed, how it will be collected and how presented (Garland, 1994, p. 21). Hansen offers an interesting perspective on what he calls the teacher's moral style by looking at tone of voice and body language in the teacher's responses to pupils and what pupils (and observing mentor) can learn from it about the teacher's values (see Hansen, 1993). Once more these processes are equally relevant to clinical supervision in health care professions, particularly because of the high level of comparability between them and teaching (see, for example, Benner, 1982).

Discussion with the student will enable sense to be made of observation and will allow the supervisor to draw the student to theorize about or reflect upon it, to enable the student to investigate it, or to make sense of the student's written work about it. Discussion can take a number of forms, most of which involve the student in reflection upon practice. (Strands of reflection (see above, p. 136) might be of use here as might also the questions in Table 7.1 above, and/or a detailed focus on critical incidents in order to investigate moral awareness, ability to theorize, the success of improvisation or other aspects of professional artistry.) Tripp (1993) provides extensive details on the use of critical incidents and James (1989) describes the important distinction between dialogue and negotiation in discussing the supervisor's assessment of the student.

Students' writing can also give a clear idea of how they make sense of practice, reflect and theorize. In clinical supervision the most appropriate form of writing to assess the sense students make of practice is the use of *portfolios and profiles* (see below). *Reflective diaries and/or journals* can also be used when spread over the total time that the student is in the clinical placement, thus facilitating the student's understanding of the experience as a whole.

In addition, the important dimension of *investigating practice* can be assessed via *reflective diaries/journals*. The processes of investigation provide a means of learning about practice-wide and profession-wide issues, and for which supervisors may be asked to help provide data, and/or contribute to the student's learning process. Indeed this process provides a major item of evidence about the student's abilities to investigate practice. Investigating practice can also be an aspect of an episode of practice, and the supervisor can contribute to this. Using supervisors to collect specific data about an episode of practice as part of this process can make an important contribution to investigating practice (see Haggar, Burn and McIntyre, 1993). Indeed, devising the observation strategies and focuses for the supervisor provides both a useful professional challenge to the student and offers evidence to the supervisor of the level of the student's thinking about investigating practice.

There is much that could be said about portfolios and profiles, and they are clearly important for assessment of reflective practice. But, it is vital to be clear about the distinctions between them, particularly because of the introduction of the use of professional profiles in a number of professions, including the very significant adoption of them as the means of maintaining professional registration in the nursing context, in the Post Registration Education and Practice (PREP) requirements introduced by the UKCC.

A *portfolio* is a collection of evidence/data on the writer's professional development. It is about self-evaluation. It is educational rather than administrative. It helps the writer to be reflective about professional practice. It is a means whereby the learner constructs his or her personal understandings. It is a learning tool. Some would wish to maintain that the portfolio is essentially a private document, owned by the writer and in which the writer can be free to explore and comment about professional things without fear of them being made public. A portfolio needs to be constructed over a reasonable period of time. Some argue that having a 'critical friend' can help these reflective processes. Some argue that this very process is itself rather problematic (see Golby and Appleby, 1995). A critical friend is intended to be one who will listen and reflect back to you the ideas, points, comments you make and helps you to become clearer about what you are saying. A supervisor might well operate as a critical friend, although the role is not easily compatible with that of formal assessor. Indeed, it may be more appropriate to set up pairings of students who work together in this way. However, the quality of what a student as critical friend can offer is variable, and although one strategy is to try to structure the roles so that even weaker students can be of some use to their colleagues, some may comment: 'With a critical friend who needs enemies?'.

By contrast to the portfolio, *a profile* is a summary or documentary history of a person's professional development. The UKCC (1995b), within the context of supervision of qualified practitioners, define a profile as 'a flexible comprehensive account of [the practitioner's] professional development and how it is to be achieved'. They go on to state that 'rather than simply recording achievements, [the practitioner's] profile is created by a continuing process which involves reflecting on and recording what you learn from everyday experiences as well as from planned learning activities'. For use in assessment, the content of a profile is often dictated by, and drawn upon, as evidence for use in a *portfolio* (reflective diary or journal). As a result, it can reflect the personal and professional progress of the individual and can offer a useful means of assessing reflective practice and professional competence. As such, it usually identifies some patterns, themes, philosophies, theories and ideals. In addition, it should enable both students and practitioners to take the longer view of their career choice, to register the quality of their professionalism and to develop a professional philosophy of their own.

All these things provide important access to many of the aspects of professionalism that the supervisor is (or ought to be) trying to assess. The work of Holly (1984, 1989), and of Squirrell *et al.* (1990), gives further details of the use of portfolios, diaries, journals and profiles. Since this aspect of professional education is developing fast, colleagues seeking to adopt these approaches need to seek examples of their use for Mode 1 supervision in their own professional journals. For example in nursing, work on profiling really only began in earnest in 1995, with the implementation of legislation which requires practitioners to maintain a professional profile as part of the process of retaining their professional registration, and so it is not possible yet to comment on or to cite the comments of others on the contribution of profiling in assessing the professionalism of practitioners. However, as the UKCC argues that an important function of the profile is to 'contribute to (the practitioner's) professional development by helping [him/her] to recognize, understand and value [his/her] abilities, strengths, achievements and profiles', it seems that profiles in the future may provide a very useful source of data for assessing this particular component of practice.

The style of assessment

Instead of assessing students by means of grades, figures and levels, we suggest (as a means of assessing the other eight aspects of professionalism that are not taken account of by competency-based assessment or equivalent) a return to the style of assessment that is in keeping with a holistic approach. Accordingly, and given that it is overall repertoires that are being assessed here, we suggest that for each aspect or focus, students are simply offered an overall pass or fail, with only the fail student being offered an analysis of the detail in order to have the chance to work on the issues necessary. This is because, under our proposals, the responsibility for recognizing their strengths and weaknesses, and for investigating their own progress in specific areas, already rests with the student, and *only* those who cannot already do this would need to be told by someone else (which in itself would be evidence of failure).

We also would argue for the overall assessment in each focus to be based upon evidence of *development* throughout the supervision period, with the student being responsible for presenting this evidence, in at least three of the four modes of assessment outlined above. Where possible it is also beneficial to have more than one person make the assessment. This should not mean more than keeping careful records of these wider issues at the same time as recording assessments of competencies which are already being carried out as a requirement.

The supervisor, professional judgement and quality assessment

It remains to note that in all this, the supervisor will be exercising many of the very attributes and aspects of professionalism that are being sought of the student, perhaps particularly since the assessment of these aspects of professionalism may require processes, understandings and professional judgements that have not hitherto been exercised in this way. For example, there is some danger of conflict between the assessment and the advisory role; the supervisor will need to be able to justify assessments, and engage in a range of different sorts of discussions (reflective, evaluatory, justificatory); there will be issues about switching between the unequal power relationship between student and assessor and critical friend (see Lucas, 1991). These will require a range of negotiative skills. There may be problems with students who seek to discover and fulfil the supervisor's agenda as protection against problems of their own being discovered. There will be students who are challenged to stretch to their best by the supervisor's presence and those who find the presence of another in the practice setting a hindrance to achieving potential. All these will need to be discerned by the supervisor and will provide many opportunities for the exercise of supervisors' professional judgement and professional artistry, and, of course, there will be the inevitable need to provide a good professional model (in the general sense) of the reflective, investigative practitioner. Thus, as Smith and Alred declare in an article aptly entitled 'The impersonation of wisdom', an important aspect of the supervisor's knowledge is self-knowledge, because 'the qualities that the mentor needs are distinct and unusual, complex and rooted in the kind of person he or she is, not simply the attributes that they have' (Smith and Alred, 1993, p. 112).

As if this were not enough, there are more advanced techniques and wider issues to which the supervisor will also need to attend, as discussed in the final part of this book, particularly in the context of supervision of the qualified practitioner.

Further reading

Benner, P. (1982). Issues in competency-based testing. *Nursing Outlook*, May, 303–309.

Bridges, D., Elliott, J. and Klass, C. (1986). Performance appraisal as naturalistic enquiry: a report of the fourth Cambridge conference on educational evaluation. *Cambridge Journal of Education*, **16**, 221–233.

Davies, I. (1993). Using profiling in initial teacher education: key issues arising from experience. *Journal of Further and Higher Education*, **17**, 27–39.

Garland, P. (1994). Using competence-based assessment positively on Certificate of Education programmes. *Journal of Further and Higher Education*, **18**, 1–22.

Holly, M. (1984). *Keeping a Personal-Professional Journal*. Deakin University.

Holly, M. (1989). Perspectives on teacher appraisal and professional development. In *Rethinking Appraisal and Assessment* (H. Simons and J. Elliott, eds) pp. 100–118, Open University Press.

Smith, R. and Alred, G. (1993). The impersonation of wisdom. In *Mentoring: Perspectives on School-based Teacher Education* (D. McIntyre, H. Haggar, and M. Wilkin, eds) pp. 103–116, Kogan Page.

Stronach, I. (1989). A critique of the 'new assessment': from currency to carnival. In *Rethinking Appraisal and Assessment* (H. Simons and J. Elliott, eds) pp. 161–179, Open University Press.

United Kingdom Central Council for Nursing, Midwifery and Health Visiting (1995b). *Prep and You*. UKCC.

Part Three

*Quality clinical supervision:
the wider responsibilities*

8

Clinical supervision for professional education: wider issues

Introduction

Previous chapters have highlighted some of the complexities of the processes of clinical supervision, have examined some contrasting approaches to it and have argued for the need for supervisors to move away from the intellectually impoverished technical–rational (TR) view of supervision in order that quality professional competence may be developed through supervision. The professional education approach to clinical supervision, which we have argued for throughout this book, is grounded in a philosophy of reflective practice. Here the supervisor's responsibilities lie not only in overseeing and developing the skills of the supervisee, and also in inducting him or her into the processes of exercising his or her own professional judgement and investigating and refining his or her practice, but also in initiating the student practitioner into (or further developing the professional in respect of) *membership of a profession.*

We would argue that these imperatives highlight some of the wider issues of supervision which need to be addressed if it is to have any chance of being truly educative and long-lasting. Most importantly, such demands indicate that supervision is an *integral* part of (rather than a separate and lesser aspect of) a high level process of preparing and developing professionals. Indeed McLaughlin (1994, p. 156) argues that practice is ' inseparable from the critique of that practice through the critical study of general principles'. Further, the move to locate the education of health care professionals within higher education, itself indicates an intention to:

> engage [them] in a properly intellectual study of the activity they are engaged in, since it is not possible to practise that activity effectively without learning at the same time to reflect critically on practice (Kelly, 1993, p. 130).

Although Scott (1995) indicates that there are now twenty different types of higher education provision in Britain, and Schuller (1995) demonstrates clearly that what counts as a university is now a highly debatable issue, we would argue with Kelly that the role of a university is:

> not only to permit, but also to promote the process of continuous questioning – of challenge, critique, dialogue, debate – which is the only route to the continued development of human knowledge and understanding (Kelly, 1993, p. 128).

All this raises questions about what should be considered as components and characteristics of quality clinical supervision.

One of the most comprehensive lists of criteria for and enlightened approaches to fieldwork education can be found in the COT's 'comprehensive and balanced criteria expected of fieldwork educators'. It contains the following list of headings, under which it offers extensive detail: performs as a professional; performs as a manager; enables learning; supports and counsels; evaluates and assesses (COT, 1994, section 8). Yet even here there is an emphasis on skills and performance, and there is no real sense of an attempt to develop critical thinking, or of the supervisor seeing, or helping the supervisee to see, beyond the placement.

By contrast, we would argue that supervisors need to consider the implications of the wider context in which the supervision takes place, and need to take seriously the problems about relating experiences in a specific placement to the wider professional education of the supervisee. This incudes taking account of and thinking analytically and critically about the present day organizational philosophy of the National Health Service or the ethos of the alternative sector; the aims of professional education; the context of higher education; and the demands of accountability and its related need to demonstrate the quality of provision. These matters raise further issues about the educational and preparational needs of supervisors if they are to work in the way proposed in this book.

This final chapter, then, attempts to address these wider issues of clinical supervision. First it considers some issues highlighted by the introduction of Mode 2 supervision in nurse education; secondly it discusses the broader issues the supervisor needs to address and the wider responsibilities he or she needs to take on, and thirdly it turns to the educational needs of the supervisor, and how to provide for quality clinical supervision. The final section then provides the individual supervisor with an agenda from which to review and re-examine the attributes required of a quality supervisor and considers the implications of this for the practice setting.

Mode 2 supervision: issues for clinical supervisors

In most professions, until recently, the role of the clinical supervisor was to work with students on course – whether the students were attempting to join a profession or were already qualified practitioners. This we have called Mode 1 supervision. But now, moves have begun in many health care professions (often as a result of pressures from quality assurance and control) to introduce the term supervision for activities that in professions like teaching are categorized as staff or professional development. It is to this Mode 2 supervision which we now turn. It might be broadly characterized in the following extract from a COT document which defines supervision for occupational therapy as:

> a system for assuring high quality occupational therapy service to the consumer. Supervision is a professional activity which is required at a number of levels, each characterized by a range of tasks. Firstly it is essential in the planning and delivery of a total programme to an organization or client group. Secondly it may be centred on the management of a group of staff and the organization of workloads. Thirdly it is a professional relationship which ensures good standards of practice and encourages professional development. [In this last] . . . it is a line relationship concerning accountability and responsibility for work carried out (COT, 1990, p. 1).

There are, COT says, many kinds of supervision. It is applicable to all types and grades of staff working with consumers. It is interesting to note that even in a profession which is very aware of educational matters for staff, the professional development role comes third only and that much of the language of the statement as a whole is drawn from management rather than education. In similar language, this document also offers a list of supervisory activities and a definition of supervisor as a recognized OT who has the responsibility for professional development of the personnel assigned and for a particular OT service. Duties include facilitating the treatment goals of the service in line with the standards adopted by the employing agent, supervising work procedures of assigned staff and improving quality of the OT service by encouraging increased competency of personnel.

In order to enable readers to consider the issues relating to Mode 2 supervision, we give below an account of recent formal developments of Mode 2 supervision in nursing. Members of other professions may wish to use it to help them consider their own profession's position, and Task 8.1 is intended to help them in this.

The introduction of the concept of clinical supervision to support the development of *qualified* staff represents a watershed in the nursing

---

**Task 8.1 Points for reflection
– for all health care professionals other than nurses**

As you read the account below, consider the following:

• How does your profession define supervision, and how is it seen as relating to clinical (or fieldwork) supervision?
• How does your profession regard (define?) professional development? (How does this differ from appraisal?)
• What provision/structure is there currently in your profession for the further development of qualified practitioners?
• What is the recent history of support and development for qualified practitioners in your profession?
• Ought there to be differences (of kind or of emphasis) between Mode 1 and Mode 2 supervision in respect of the role and of the skills and abilities of the supervisor? (And if so, what ought these to be?)
• Is there, or ought there to be, a code of conduct for supervisors in your profession? (If there is, what are its key tenets?)
• How might clinical supervision of the Mode 2 kind be protected from becoming a managerial tool rather than an educational one?

---

profession. Swain (1995, p. 28) argues that the profession has been 'notoriously bad at supporting staff, and nurses are often reluctant to request support believing it unreasonable to want or even express the need for it'. This highlights the issue of what the relationship should be between clinical supervisor and the supervisee. Obviously supervision needs to be carried out in a supportive environment but it is also much more than simply giving support. This in turn raises questions about the counselling role of the supervisor and the extent to which counselling skills are required of the supervisor. Such issues indicate the potential for the use and misuse of clinical supervision (particularly in supervision offered to qualified practitioners) and this also emphasizes the importance of ethical matters in respect of supervision.

In nursing, both the supervisee and the supervisor are bound by the professional code of conduct (UKCC, 1992b), which provides protection of the interests of patients, clients and practitioners, but it may be that the supervisory process requires much clearer guidelines, particularly in relation to the nature of supervision, the question of responsibility and issues of competence. Indeed Swain (1995) notes that trusts and units within the NHS organizational structure have been recommended to draw up a code of ethics and practice in the context of supervision using the code of ethics provided by the British Association of Counselling as a guideline. This is particularly relevant in situations where the relationship between the supervisor and supervisee breaks down either because the one feels unable to supervise or the other feels inadequately supervised. These points about the use and misuse of supervision, although discussed in the context of qualified practitioners, might equally be significant in student supervision, where in addition the supervisor plays a direct gatekeeping role during the supervisory process.

Questions about the use and misuse of supervision also highlight the relationship between clinical and management supervision. In the case studies provided in the publication by Kohner (1994), examples are given where the manager in the unit has responsibility for the supervision of staff within that unit. In these examples the supervisors acknowledge the complexity of carrying out a dual role but argue that it contributes to the supervisory process since it allows practitioners to 'be given instant feedback on their day to day practice' (Kohner, 1994, p. 10). Swain (1995), however, argues that perceived links between clinical supervision and management supervision have created anxiety for practitioners about the role of clinical supervision and, following an analysis of the different issues, this approach to supervision is not recommended as good practice for practitioners within the discipline of community health care nursing. The particular concern that there may be misuse of clinical supervision in feeding evidence to formal disciplinary processes has now been allayed (see UKCC, 1996a).

It is interesting to observe that in midwifery practice this debate is not apparent since the guidelines for the supervision of midwives make a clear link between management and clinical supervision. Evidence such as this highlights the need for supervisors to consider whether they should assume this dual responsibility, in particular because of the implications it may have not only for the supervisory process but also in creating conflict of interests. Indeed, supervisors who assume this approach have to consider whether their major responsibility is in developing practice or merely identifying poor quality of care. In addition they need to consider the extent to which clinical supervision should contribute to individual performance review (IPR) and staff appraisal. In our view, any confusion of roles is very likely to produce a conflict of interests and a compromise of quality supervision.

However, the issue is even more complex than this. For example, even where supervisors do not assume this dual responsibility, conflict of interest can also arise. Three major factors have been identified in contributing to this process. The first of these is time management, since clinical supervisors generally retain a clinical role and must decide how to allocate their time to different responsibilities. Another important factor is the quality and nature of the relationship with the supervisee. Miller (cited in Swain, 1995) describes the supervisor as the centre of a triangle consisting of the practitioner, client (or patient) and the agency. Tensions may be created within this triad because of the different needs and approaches to care and the supervisor will need to manage them in order to offer quality supervision. Such tensions may result from a different emphasis on practice priorities, particularly where the supervisor is committed to the integration of theory and practice and considers this concept fundamental to providing quality supervision. Yet a further factor which can contribute to a conflict of interests is the creation of a purchaser-provider philosophy in the provision of health care. In our view it is essential that supervisors understand and consider the implications of this.

The development of a purchaser-provider philosophy in the organization of the NHS has created an internal market where purchasers have the responsibility for identifying the health needs and requirements of their populations and providers have the responsibility of providing services to meet these identified needs both in the hospital and community context. The ability of purchasers to change the provider with whom they place the contract has introduced a level of competition previously unknown in the NHS. Supporters of this approach to the organization of care argue that the introduction of competition should improve the quality of care and service provision. The need for support for clinical supervision within this political climate from the professional regulatory body (the UKCC) has been identified by executive nurses working in provider units in order that the significance for high quality care is recognized by purchasers and providers (Smith, 1995). Indeed Swain (1995) argues that no purchaser should consider contracting services from a provider unit where clinical supervision is not an integral component of the provision of that unit.

Where clinical supervision has been introduced within the business plans of providers it raises questions, in our view, about the control that supervisors have over the content and approach of the supervisory process. The likelihood is that many providers will opt for an approach to supervision that is grounded in a model of TR rather than reflective practice since TR comes from a philosophy that fits within the current political context of the NHS. This calls into doubt the extent to which supervisors may be able to carry out quality supervision and also clouds the responsibilities of the individual supervisor within the organizational setting. Such confusions are more likely to become entrenched, and the less educational will become their work, the more supervisors and those they work with accept uncritically these ideas and the imposition of these conditions. It is an argument in itself for nurses to engage in more critical analysis and reflection on their practice and its context.

The broader issues for and wider responsibilities of the supervisor

Supervisors who seek to facilitate both students and qualified practitioners in achieving their potential in professional development need to consider the wider issues of professional education, rather than merely the supervision of practice skills. The arguments outlined below provide a rationale for focusing the supervisory process on the wider issues involved in the characteristics and components of professional education.

First, skills alone provide no basis for professional activity since the supervision of skills alone offers no insight as to when, why and how to use the skills. In addition professional practice is not an activity in which processes and outcomes can be predetermined. Secondly, the work of the practice setting cannot provide adequate preparation for effective professional development. There is no doubt that it provides the student or the qualified practitioner with a vast range of perspectives on the practice of that particular setting, by focusing on one or two ways of carrying out that particular practice activity. But it cannot do justice to the complexities of practice, nor to the demands of being a member of a profession – in particular the consequences of the organizational pressures of professional practice and the demands of and responsibilities to society, which are essential components of professional life.

In fact supervision which focuses on practical skills and the highly individual context and specific expertise faces some very difficult questions about its value, generalizability, relevance and significance in contributing to the professional development of practitioners, if it is to enable them to operate effectively in different conditions and on different occasions. Indeed it is essential that the supervisee has the chance to review assumptions and develop a broadly informed, critical approach to practice, which is unlikely to occur in the situation where the supervision focuses only on skills for the practice setting.

Equally, however, reflection on practice is not, of itself, necessarily of value if used regardless of its informing perspectives, procedures and outcomes. Reflection used inappropriately or unsystematically can both undermine a supervisee's practice and distort understanding. Jarvis (1994) helpfully points out that *contemplation* can be characterized as the 'process of thinking about an experience and reaching a conclusion without reference to wider social reality' (Jarvis, 1994, p. 38). A way to avoid these problems is to be able to raise questions about reflection and its appropriate usage and in doing so be able to draw upon the illuminations of a range of traditions of thought and research in professional practice. Indeed a principled, reflective approach to practice (and supervision), which involves consideration of a wide range of theoretical perspectives, is an important foundation for practice for both the student and the qualified practitioner and should be a component of quality supervision. Adopting this approach to supervision allows the supervisee to gain access to a broader understanding of professional practice. It is, we believe, an important responsibility of the supervisor.

In the literature on teacher education, Fish (1995) has presented two distinct views of what teaching is about; the first of these views she describes as the unproblematic and the second as the initiation view. The unproblematic view is one that represents practice as something that is properly described in neutral language using the statutory competencies or learning outcomes and regards them as activities to be performed. The initiation view has been developed in contrast by teacher educators who, in attempting to sketch the content necessary to prepare a teacher to become a full member of the profession, have used very different language. They suggest the school should be used as the starting point for a broader professional education. By using the school as a source for investigating wider professional issues, questions can be raised about how things are done and why they are done, which leads to questions about alternative practices and their relative merits and to a consideration of the evidence being used in discussing such matters and the interests being served. The importance of understanding the activities in a particular setting as part of a *broad social practice* are highlighted.

A similar scenario is present in health care. If supervisors remain focused on the learning outcomes provided by the professional statutory body rather than considering the activities of practice in the wider context of professional practice, they will produce narrowly focused practitioners. Once again, it is clear that supervisors need to acknowledge and adopt their wider responsibilities if quality supervision is to be provided.

The contribution of theory to the understanding of students' practice and that of the supervisor is also usefully explored from within the context of education by Smith (1992). He suggests that theory is not best articulated in terms of content but in respect of what it can do for the student. He suggests that it can: challenge implicit theory (since students come with their own); show that things can be otherwise; develop a sense of what is involved in education; make professional practice interesting by opening up the diversity of perspectives and encouraging practitioners to formulate their own philosophy; create an intelligent profession. This he defines as one that reflects on practice, sees it as problematic and open to change, and is prepared to deliberate about, rather than assert or accede to, polarizing tendencies of the media. Smith goes on to argue that these matters are vital since the world of teaching is becoming increasingly complex. We would argue this interpretation of the contribution of theory to practice is equally pertinent to health care where the practice world is making increasingly complex demands on practitioners, and that this, in turn, has implications for supervision. Supervisors who adopt this interpretation of the role of theory in supervision can provide the supervisee with the opportunity for exploring the wider issues of professional practice and for investigating thoughtfully the integration of theory with practice in the reality of the practice setting.

Finally, the statutory body for nursing, the UKCC, has also contributed to the debate about the wider responsibilities of supervisors in health care generally with publications such as *The Scope of Professional Practice* (UKCC, 1992a). In contrast to the learning outcomes provided by the UKCC for the student practitioner, *The Scope of Professional Practice* adopts an approach much more like that of professional education described above. This document, which was written to meet the continually changing demands and complexities facing practitioners in everyday practice, provides a set of principles which underpin the scope of professional practice. These principles include concepts fundamental to professional education and practice, such as that which requires 'practitioners to acknowledge any limits of personal knowledge and skill and take steps to remedy any relevant deficits in order effectively and appropriately to meet the needs of patients and clients' (UKCC, 1992a, p. 6). This approach requires practitioners to consider practice in a much broader context than previously, when extended roles in practice were more clearly defined. The Department of Health, in linking the target on clinical supervision in the new strategy for nursing directly to the scope of professional practice, demonstrates the need for supervisors not only to consider the implications of this interpretation for the supervisory process, but also to accept the wider responsibilities associated with this interpretation if professional development is to be achieved amongst students and practitioners. Further examples of these wider issues can be found in the UKCC's *Guidelines for Professional Practice* (UKCC, 1996b).

In our view these wider responsibilities reinforce the essential role that reflection plays in the supervisory process. If, however, reflection is to be properly informed and systematic, the understanding which shapes that reflection must be appropriately scholarly and embedded in a critical tradition. These demands on the supervisor demonstrate the need for practitioners to receive preparation to carry out their role as supervisors.

Quality supervision: implications for the preparation of supervisors

The importance of effective preparation for supervisors is strongly supported in literature, on, for example, nursing, occupational therapy, and physiotherapy and, in all health care professions recognized by the government, there are regulations in place which ensure that some preparation of clinical supervisors is attended to. But the content and format of much of that preparation is less well defined, with different professions and different writers presenting very different opinions about it. The very terminology used to describe this preparation perhaps highlights some of the issues which need to be considered.

In physiotherapy, Standard 4 of the *Standards for Clinical Placement* lists the following as the required content of a recognized course for clinical educators: teaching skills; assessment skills, including giving feedback; an understanding of the learning process; time management skills; interpersonal skills (CSP, 1991, p. 5). Although this seems rather skills-oriented, the CSP's published guidelines on its expectations for the support of clinical educators describe two types of course, the first of which is concerned with a grounding in educational concepts. Taken together, these would suggest a concern for some matters beyond skills, and, indeed, guideline 26 (CSP, 1994) indicates that this should include teaching skills, assessment methodologies, giving and receiving constructive feedback, educational theories related to adult learning, curriculum planning, and teaching and learning styles as well as development of the reflective practitioner. But even so it is not clear how far, in *practice*, this extends to the kinds of issues we discuss.

In nursing almost all the literature either states or implies a view that learning to supervise is indeed about learning skills. Swain (1995) refers to the preparation for nursing supervision as training and states that the training should include 'counselling skills, an understanding of the supervision framework and understanding of interpersonal dynamics'. Kohner (1994, p. 39) likewise describes the preparation of supervisors as training, stating that 'all supervisors should be given opportunities to receive training and learn skills that are needed to provide supervision that is both constructive and supportive'. Although these skills are not specifically identified, examples such as counselling, management and teaching are given. Faugier and Butterworth (1993) provide a review of the preparatory needs of supervisors in nursing. In this review, although they acknowledge the need for some 'unlearning' so that the supervisor becomes more conscious of his or her supervisory role, generally the preparation is described in terms of training, but they provide no specific content, which makes it difficult to determine the extent to which this is the case.

In occupational therapy, a previous 'sequential approach' to preparing supervisors (with five course levels, many of them heavily skills-based) has now given way to placing the onus on the individual to demonstrate that he or she can fulfil the demands of the COT. These demands are still performance-related and to some extent skill-based, but they do represent (in our view) a broader understanding of this whole matter than can be found in nursing or physiotherapy.

Evidence of this is as follows. For example, the central concept now operating in OT is of 'fieldwork education'. Now COT requires that no OT should be accredited as a supervisor 'unless able to demonstrate commitment to fieldwork education [and] the skills of self-evaluation as a pre-requisite to evaluating the performance of others' and where 'evaluation' – a somewhat surprising term – is defined as 'the process of continued reflective dialogue which enables the student to develop knowledge, skills and attitudes for professional practice' (COT, 1994, p. 4). Such an approach 'involves a partnership between supervisor and student in a fieldwork setting [and] offers an opportunity for rehearsal and reflection and both complements and supplements academic studies' (COT, 1993, p. 2). Here the functions of the fieldwork educator (or fieldwork supervisor) are to be an educator and assessor, to perform as a professional concerned with the consumer; to manage self and student; to enable learning, teach, guide, facilitate, support and counsel, and to contribute actively to the evaluation and assessment of performance and competence to practice. The 'performance criteria' of a fieldwork educator are detailed under five headings: performs as a professional; performs as a manager; enables learning; supports and counsels students; and evaluates and assesses performance (COT, 1994, pp. 57–8). Supervisors are encouraged to use a professional profile to collect evidence about their own development as a supervisor under these headings, citing such evidence from the following sources: in-house practice; update/reading; written information; specific briefing; self-evaluation; student testimony; peer/manager testimony; course tutor testimony; and information relating to specific courses (COT, 1994, p. 11).

This brief analysis of the preparation considered appropriate for supervisors in nursing and physiotherapy, and (by contrast) occupational therapy, raises some significant issues which require addressing. These are: first whether training is an appropriate approach for preparation; and secondly whether an emphasis on the rather more humanistic skills of counselling (which we see particularly in nursing) will be sufficient to meet the needs of supervisors wishing to focus on their wider responsibilities in supervision.

The approach to preparation which focuses on a training model (or even a model which hands down education to passive learners) clearly reflects a model of supervision grounded in a philosophy of TR. Further, such preparation for a passive supervisor is likely in turn to produce a biddable and uncritical workforce. For example, an emphasis on training implies that the focus of the supervisory process is on promulgating the policies and procedures considered by the trainers to be appropriate for that professional practice. If, however, the approach to supervision adopted in the practice setting is to be the model of professional education advocated earlier in this chapter, then training supervisors in skills (like those of counselling, management and even teaching), will not prepare them for it. Indeed, if the student or practitioner is to reach his or her potential in professional development, the preparation will need to focus on the much wider issues of professional practice and include the *understanding* necessary for coping with the complexities of the practice situation.

The second question to be considered is the extent to which preparation focused on the counselling skills of the supervisor is any more adequate as an approach to tackling the wider issues. Obviously it is important that the supervisor and supervisee have an effective working relationship otherwise the quality of the supervisory process is likely to be affected. An understanding of the processes involved in counselling and the ability to implement these skills in practice will enhance the supervisory process. However, we would wish to argue that training in counselling skills alone will not produce quality supervision, but that skills in facilitating reflection on practice are essential.

Part of our evidence for maintaining this comes from research we carried out earlier, which demonstrated the difficulty experienced by practitioners working as clinical teachers in helping students to reflect on their practice (Fish, Twinn and Purr, 1991). Generally the level of dialogue between the practitioner and the student practitioners was merely descriptive and therefore did not lead to any critical analysis or interpretations of practice as illustrated in the Strands of reflection in Chapter 5. Thus we would argue that in order to promote effective supervision for both students and practitioners alike it is essential that strategies such as Strands of reflection are addressed during the preparatory period. Readers should now attempt Task 8.2.

In planning a supervision course you may also wish to think about how experiences from practice can be utilized and how these experiences may be transferred to other learning situations; how the practice setting is understood as part of a broad social practice; how this may set up conflicts between differing traditions; and how access to broader understanding involves reviewing assumptions which have been previously held. These issues are particularly relevant if the supervisor is to take on the wider responsibilities of clinical supervision. What is perhaps less debatable is that the course should include discussion on

---

Task 8.2. Planning a supervision course
(with a colleague or colleagues)

Plan a short modular course for clinical supervisors.

1 In planning this course you will need to consider:
   • your philosophy of clinical supervision
   • the kind of professional you want to develop (a critical thinker/ someone just able to meet the demands of the job/ a member of the profession?)
   • how you define professional development for practitioners and how that might relate to their initial preparation course.
2 What should be included in the course, and at what level? (What does a supervisor need to know and what should he or she be able to do?)
   • theory/practice; practice-focused skills; educational strategies; educational understanding; consideration of reflection and professional judgement; professional issues.
   • what makes up practitioners' professional knowledge?
3 What teaching, learning and assessment strategies will you adopt?
4 Would you include a period of supervision?
   • If so what would this involve?

---

the characteristics and components of the quality supervisor. The final section of this chapter provides supervisors with the opportunity of considering those attributes and characteristics as well as the impact of clinical supervision on the practice setting in which the clinical supervisor works.

Quality supervision: a way forward

In determining the way forward for quality supervision there are two major factors to consider: first the supervisor as a person and secondly the impact of clinical supervision on the clinical setting. The attributes and characteristics of quality supervision have been addressed at various places in previous chapters. The points for discussion listed in Task 8.3 provide an overview of the attributes and characteristics of the quality supervisor.

What attributes are involved in being a quality supervisor? Like all educational questions the answer will be value-based. Readers might like to consider the main values underlying the following list:

• being a learner and seeker and being willing to tackle new ideas and practices

<hr>

Task 8.3 Points for consideration

1 Reconsider the agenda you made at the start of the book, and check whether you have achieved what you intended.
2 Review the main areas of your learning and trace your changing ideas. What has caused you to make these changes?
3 Jot down the key characteristics of a supervisor that make for quality supervision.
4 Compare your list with the list below.

<hr>

- being willing to open up practice and knowing how, when and to what end to do this with students and practitioners so that they can think critically about theirs
- being able to offer constructive debriefing which leads ultimately to student or practitioner self-assessment
- being able to discuss and demonstrate a variety of practice strategies and to cope with the unexpected
- being able to demonstrate that one's practice is principled
- being able to enunciate some of those principles
- being willing to open up to discussion on one's ideas
- being aware of the value-base of one's work
- being able to pin-point and explain the underlying theories of one's practice
- being someone who reflects on practice and is self-critical
- being someone who investigates practice with a view to refining it
- understanding the problematic nature of issues
- being able to lead students and practitioners to reflective theorizing
- knowing what one is and is not sure of, and saying so openly
- being tolerant, open-minded and able to live with one's uncertainties
- being happy to enable others to find their own ways of practising
- being able to cope with both the role of enabler and role of supervisor
- being aware of the moral dimension to supervision
- knowing about the wider dimensions of professional practice and being able to see it holistically
- being a reader of professional literature
- being flexible and able to cope with the wide range of roles demanded in supervision (interviewing, teaching, investigating, reflecting, counselling, gate-keeping).

In short, perhaps, these might be summarized as having suitable personal qualities and taking a principled approach to practice. This leaves us with the final question: what sort of impact might this whole approach to supervision have on the practice setting?

The impact of supervision on the practice setting

The demands that clinical supervisors make on the practice setting are usually considerable, particularly in terms of staff time and levels of stress, but any local difficulties ought to be far outweighed by the extensive benefits gained. Put in a nutshell, the activity of supervision and of seeking to become a quality supervisor is a major staff development activity. If it has not already begun, the time to begin it is now. One possible beginning might be by staff simply sharing the experiences of reflection on and investigation of their own practice, and experimenting in explaining to each other the principles underlying their practice, their espoused theories and their theories-in-use. (Some of the tasks offered in early chapters above might be helpful here; see also McIntyre (1994).) Then, assuming that any member of the practice setting who works in any way with a student is a supervisor, one approach to looking at involvement of the whole practice setting is to discuss:

- some attributes involved in being a supervisor
- what knowledge is involved in being a supervisor?
- what, in the ethos of the practice setting, provides for these things? (What enables – or would enable – the practice setting to become a more reflective community?)
- what expertise is already available, and where is it?
- what staff development provision is now needed?

Such questions lead to the major questions of whether the practice setting is a learning practice setting and also a reflective practice setting, whether all its staff can be characterized as, and whether all its strategies are aimed at, seeking to improve supervision and practice through personal development. We would argue that this ought to be so.

There is always more to do and more to learn. Quality in patient and client care is not achieved by decree nor by striving to reach standards set by others which are frequently raised before we can reach them. Rather it is achieved by the endless pursuit, by each practitioner, of greater understanding and better practice, and the clinical supervisor's role in this is, quite simply, central.

References

Abbott, P. and Sapsford, R. (1992). *Research into Practice: a Reader for Nurses and the Caring Professions*. Open University Press.

Acton, G., Irving, B. and Hopkins, B. (1991). Theory – testing research: building the science. *Advanced Nursing Science*, **14**, 52–61.

Alexander, R. (1990). Partnership in initial teacher education: confronting the issues. In *Partnership in Initial Teacher Training* (M. Booth, J. Furlong and M. Wilkin, eds) pp. 59–73. Cassell.

Alsop, A. (1993). The developmental model of skill acquisition in fieldwork. *British Journal of Occupational Therapy*, **56**, 7–12.

Alsop, A. and Ryan, S. (1996). *Making the Most of Fieldwork Education: a Practical Guide*. Chapman and Hall.

Anning, A., Broadhead, P., Busher, H. *et al.* (1990). *Using Video-recordings for Teacher Professional Development*. University of Leeds.

Argyris, C. and Schön, D. A. (1974). *Theory in Practice*. Jossey Bass.

Ashcroft, K. and Foreman-Peck, L. (1994). *Managing Teaching and Learning in Further and Higher Education*. Falmer Press.

Ashworth, P. D. and Saxton, J. (1990). On competence. *Journal of Further and Higher Education*, **14**, 3–25.

Austin, C. and Herbert, S. (1995). Clinical guidelines: Should we be worried? *British Journal of Occupational Therapy*, **58**, 481–484.

Barker, P. (1992). Psychiatric nursing. In *Clinical Supervision and Mentorship in Nursing* (T. Butterworth and J. Faugier, eds) pp. 65–79. Chapman and Hall.

Bell, J., Bush, T. and Fox, A. *et al.* (1984). *Conducting Small-scale Investigations in Educational Management*. Harper and Row.

Benner, P. (1982). Issues in competency-based testing. *Nursing Outlook*, May, 303–309.

Benner, P. (1984). *From Novice to Expert*. Addison-Wesley.

Benner, P. and Wrubel, J. (1989). *The Primacy of Caring: Stress and Coping in Health and Illness*. Addison-Wesley.

Benett, I. and Danczak, A. (1994). Terminal care: improving teamwork in primary care using significant event analysis. *European Journal of Cancer Care*, **3**, 54–57.

Bennett, E. (1994). Is clinical audit action research? *Educational Action Research*, **2**, 415–421.

Bernard, L. A. and Walsh, M. (1990). *Leadership: the Key to the Professionalization of Nursing*, 2nd edn. C. V. Mosby Co.

Bishop, V. and Butterworth, T. (1994). *Proceedings of the Clinical Supervision Conference*. NHSE.

Bond, S. (1993). Experimental research in nursing: necessary but not sufficient. In *Nursing: Art and Science* (A. Kitson, ed.) pp. 94–110. Chapman and Hall.

Boud, D. and Walker, D. (1991). In the midst of experience: developing a model to aid learners and facilitators. Unpublished paper presented at Empowerment through Experiential Learning: Explorations of Good Practice: A National Conference at the University of Surrey, 16–18 July 1991.

Boud, D., Keogh, R. and Walker, D. (eds) (1985). *Reflection: Turning Experience into Learning*. Kogan Page.

Bradley, C. P. (1992). Turning anecdotes into data – the critical incident technique. *Family Practitioner: an International Journal*, **9**, 98–103.

Bridges, D., Elliott, J. and Klass, C. (1986). Performance appraisal as naturalistic enquiry: a report of the fourth Cambridge conference on educational evaluation. *Cambridge Journal of Education*, **16**, 221–233.

British Medical Association (1993). *Complementary Medicine: New Approaches to Good Practice*. BMA.

Broadfoot, P. (ed.) (1986). *Profiles and Records of Achievement: a Review of Issues and Practice*. Holt Education.

Broadhead, P. (1987). A blue-print for the good teacher? The HMI/DES model of good primary practice. *British Journal of Educational Studies*, **35**, 57–71.

Broadhead, P. (1990). Perceptual issues in the use of video in educational research. In *Using Video-recordings for Teacher Professional Development* (A. Anning, P. Broadhead, H. Busher, eds) pp. 124–139. University of Leeds.

Bruni, N. (1991). Nursing knowledge: processes of production. In *Towards a Discipline of Nursing* (G. Gray and R. Pratt, eds) pp. 171–190. Churchill Livingstone.

Bullough, R. and Gitlin, A. (1994). Challenging teacher education as training: four propositions. *Journal of Education for Teaching*, **20**, 67–82.

Bulman, C. (1994). Exemplars of reflection: other people can do it, why not you too? In *Reflective Practice in Nursing* (A. Palmer, S. Burns and C. Bulman, eds) pp. 131–154. Blackwell Scientific Publications.

Burke, J. (ed.) (1989). *Competency-based Education and Training*. Falmer Press.

Butterworth, T. (1992). Clinical supervision as an emerging idea in nursing. In *Clinical Supervision and Mentorship in Nursing* (T. Butterworth and J. Faugier, eds) pp. 3–17. Chapman and Hall.

Butterworth, T. and Faugier, J. (eds) (1992). *Clinical Supervision and Mentorship in Nursing*. Chapman and Hall.

Calderhead, J. (ed.) (1988). *Teachers' Professional Learning*. Falmer Press.

Calderhead, J. (1989). Reflective teaching and teacher education. *Teaching and Teacher Education*, **5**, 43–51.

Cameron-Jones, M. (1991). *Training Teachers: a Practical Guide*. Scottish Council for Research in Education.

Carr, D. (1993). Questions of competence. *British Journal of Educational Studies*, **41**, 253–271.

Carr, W. (1987). What is an educational practice? *Journal of Philosophy of Education*, **21**, 163–175.

Carr, W. and Kemmis, S. (1986). *Becoming Critical: Education, Knowledge and Action Research*. Falmer Press.

Chartered Society of Physiotherapists (1991). *Standards for Clinical Education Placements*. CSP.

Chartered Society of Physiotherapists (1994). Guideline 26: *Guidelines for Good Practice in the Education of Clinical Educators*. CSP.

Chief Nursing Officer Professional Letter (1994). Clinical supervision: for the nursing and health visiting professions. *CNO* **94 (5)**. Department of Health.

Chown, A. and Last, J. (1993). Can the NCVQ model be used for teacher training? *Journal of Further and Higher Education*, **17**, 15–26.

Clark, C. M. (1988). Asking the right questions about teacher preparation: contributions of research on teacher thinking. *Educational Researcher*, **17**, 5–12.

College of Occupational Therapists (1990). *Standards, Policies and Proceedings: Students on Supervision in Occupational Therapy*. (SSP100) COT.

College of Occupational Therapists (1993). *Guidelines for Assessing the Quality of the Fieldwork Education of Occupational Therapy Students*. (SPP165) COT.

College of Occupational Therapists (1994). *Recommended Requirements for the Accreditation of Fieldwork Educators*. (SPP166) COT.

Council for Complementary and Alternative Medicine (1993). *CCAM: The Council for Complementary and Alternative Medicine*. CCAM.

Council for National Academic Awards (1992). *Profiling in Higher Education: Guidelines for the Development and Use of Profiling Schemes*. Council for National Academic Awards (CNAA).

Council for Professions Supplementary to Medicine (1995). *Who We Are and What We Do*. CPSM.

Culshaw, H. (1995). Evidence-based practice for sale? *British Journal of Occupational Therapy*, **58**, 233.

Dalley, G. (1993). The ideological foundations of informal care. In *Nursing: Art and Science* (A. Kitson, ed.) pp. 11–24. Chapman and Hall.

Darbyshire, P. (1991). Telling stories: nursing reflections. *Nursing Times*, **87**, 27–30.

Darbyshire, P. (1994). Skilled expert practice: Is it 'all in the mind'? A response to English's critique of Benner's Novice to Expert Model. *Journal of Advanced Nursing*, **19**, 755–761.

Davidson, L. and Lucas, J. H. (1995). Multiprofessional education in the under-graduate professions curriculum: observations from Adelaide, Linköping and Salford. *Journal of Interprofessional Care*, **9**, 163–176.

Davies, I. (1993). Using profiling in initial teacher education. *Journal of Further and Higher Education*, **17**, 227–239.

Department of Health (1989). *A Strategy of Nursing*. DoH Nursing Division.

Department of Health (1992). *The Health of the Nation: A Strategy for Health in England*. Her Majesty's Stationery Office (HMSO).

Department of Health (1993). *Targeting Practice: the Contribution of Nurses, Midwives and Health Visitors*. DoH.

Dewey, J. (1933). *How We Think*. D. C. Heath & Co.

Dreyfus, H. L. and Dreyfus, S. E. (1986). *Mind Over Machine*. Free Press.

Dunne, E. and Dunne, R. (1993). The purpose and impact of school-based work: the class-teacher's role. In *Learning to Teach* (N. Bennett and C. Carré, eds) pp. 135–148. Routledge.

Dunne, R. and Harvard, G. (1993). A model of teaching and its implications for mentoring. In *Mentoring: Perspectives on School-based Teacher Education* (D. McIntyre, H. Haggar and M. Wilkin, eds) pp. 117–129. Kogan Page.

Edwards, A. and Knight, P. (eds) (1995). *Assessing Competence in Higher Education*. Kogan Page.

English, I. (1993). Intuition as a function of the expert nurse: a critique of Benner's novice to expert model. *Journal of Advanced Nursing*, **18**, 387–393.

English National Board (1985). *New Outline Curriculum – Teaching and Assessing in Clinical Practice Course 998*, Circular 1985/36/BI. ENB.

English National Board (1994). *Supervision of Midwives*. ENB.

English National Board (1995). *Creating Life-long Learners Partnerships for Care*. ENB.

Eraut, M. (1989). Initial teacher training and the NVQ model. In *Competency-based Education and Training* (J. Burke, ed.) pp. 171–185. Falmer Press.

Eraut, M. (1995). Schön shock: a case for reframing reflection-in-action? *Teachers and Training: Theory and Practice*, **1**, 9–23.

Evans, M. (1991). Professional ethics and reflective practice: a moral analysis. In *Towards a Discipline of Nursing* (G. Gray and R. Pratt, eds) pp. 309–335. Churchill Livingstone.

Faugier, J. and Butterworth, T. (1993). *Clinical Supervision: a Position Paper*. University of Manchester.

Fielding, S. J. and Sharp, G. J. (1995). Competences: their development and value in contemporary health care education. The experience of the osteopaths. *Complementary Therapies in Medicine*, **3**, 42–45.

Fish, D. (1989). *Learning Through Practice in Initial Teacher Training*. Kogan Page.

Fish, D. (1995). *Quality Mentoring for Student Teachers: a Principled Approach to Practice*. David Fulton.

Fish, D. and Purr, B. (1991). *An Evaluation of Practice-based Learning in Continuing Education in Nursing, Midwifery and Health Visiting*. ENB.

Fish, D., Twinn, S. and Purr, B. (1990). *How to Enable Learning Through Professional Practice*. West London Press.

Fish, D., Twinn, S. and Purr, B. (1991). *Promoting Reflection: Improving the Supervision of Practice in Health Visiting and Initial Teacher Training*. West London Institute.

Fisher, F. (1995). Complementary medicine: new approaches to good practice. *Complementary Therapies in Medicine*, **3**, 5.

Ford, P. and Walsh, M. (1994). *New Rituals for Old*. Butterworth-Heinemann.

Freidson, E. (1994). *Professionalism Reborn: Theory, Prophecy and Policy*. Polity Press in association with Blackwell.

Garland, P. (1994). Using competence-based assessment positively on Certificate in Education programmes. *Journal of Further and Higher Education*, **18**, 16–22.

Gilroy, P. (1993). Reflections on Schön: an epistemological critique and a practical alternative. *International Analysis of Teacher Education: Journal of Education for Teaching*, **19**, 83–89.

Golby, M. (1989). Teachers and their research. In *Quality in Teaching* (W. Carr, ed.) pp. 163–172. Falmer Press.

Golby, M. (1993a). Editorial comments. In *A Reader provided for M.Ed. Students at Exeter University*, (limited publication). Fair Way Publications.

Golby, M. (1993b). *Case Study as Educational Research*. Fair Way Publications.

Golby, M. and Appleby, R. (1995). Reflective practice through critical friendship: some possibilities. *Cambridge Journal of Education*, **25**, 149–160.

Goodyear, R. (1992). The inservice curriculum for teachers: a review of policy, control and balance. *British Journal of Educational Studies*, **40**, 379–399.

Gray, J. and Forsstrom, S. (1991). Generating theory from practice: the reflective technique. In *Towards a Discipline of Nursing* (G. Gray and R. Pratt, eds) pp. 355–372. Churchill Livingstone.

Griffiths, M. and Tann, S. (1992). Using reflective practice to link personal and public theories. *Journal of Education for Teaching*, **18**, 69–84.

Griffiths, P. (1995). Progress in measuring nursing outcomes. *Journal of Advanced Nursing*, **21**, 1092–1100.

Haggar, H., Burn, K. and McIntyre, D. (1993). *The School Mentor Handbook*. Kogan Page.

Hansen, D. (1993). The moral importance of the teacher's style. *Journal of Curriculum Studies*, 25, 397–421.

Hartley, D. (1992). *Teacher Appraisal: a Policy Analysis*. Scottish Academic Press.

Hartley, D. (1993). Confusion in teacher education: a post-modern condition. *International Analysis of Teacher Education: Journal of Education for Teaching*, **19**, 83–89.

Harvey, L., Mason, S. and Ward, R. (1995). *The Role of Professional Bodies in Higher Education Quality Monitoring*. Centre for Research in Quality, University of Central England.

Hawkins, P. and Shohet, R. (1989). *Supervision in the Helping Professions*. Open University Press.

Health Visitors Association (1995). Clinical Supervision. *Health Visitor*, **68**, 28–31.

Higgs, J. (1992). Managing clinical education: the educational manager and the self-directed learner. *Physiotherapy*, **78**, 822–828.

Higgs, J. and Jones, L. (1995). *Clinical Reasoning in the Health Professions*. Butterworth-Heinemann.

Hitchcock, G. (1989). *Profiles and Profiling: a Practical Introduction*. Longman.

Holly, M. L. (1984). *Keeping a Personal-professional Journal*. Deakin University.

Holly, M. L. (1989). Perspectives on teacher appraisal and professional development. In *Rethinking Appraisal and Assessment* (H. Simons and J. Elliott, eds) pp. 100–118. Open University Press.

Hopkins, D. (1985). *A Teacher's Guide to Classroom Research*. Open University Press.

Hopkins, D. and Reid, K. (eds) (1985). *Rethinking Teacher Education*. Croom Helm.

Hoyle, E. (1974). Professionality, professionalism and the control of teaching. *London Educational Review*, **3**, 13–18.

James, M. (1989). Negotiation and dialogue in student assessment and teacher appraisal. In *Rethinking Appraisal and Assessment* (H. Simons and J. Elliott, eds) pp. 149–160. Open University Press.

Jarvis, P. (1983). *Professional Education*. Croom Helm.

Jarvis, P. (1994). Learning practical knowledge. *Journal of Further and Higher Education*, **18**, 31–43.

Johns, C. (1993). Professional supervision. *Journal of Nursing Management*, **1**, 9–18.

Johns, C. (1994). Guided reflection. In *Reflective Practice in Nursing* (A. Palmer, S. Burns and C. Bulman, eds) pp. 110–130. Blackwell Scientific Publications.

Johns, C. (1995). The value of reflective practice for nursing. *Journal of Clinical Nursing*, **4**, 23–30.

Jones, L. and Moore, R. (1993). Education, competence and the control of expertise. *British Journal of Sociology of Education*, **14**, 385–397.

Kelly, A. V. (1993). Education as a field of study in a university: challenge, critique, dialogue, debate. *Journal of Education for Teaching*, **19**, 125–139.

Kenny, W. W. and Grotelleuschen, A. (1984). Making the case for case study, *Journal of Curriculum Studies*, **16**, 37–51.

Kenworthy, N. and Nicklin, P. (1989). *Teaching and Assessing in Nursing Practice*. Scutari Press.

Kohner, N. (1994). *Clinical Supervision in Practice*. King's Fund Centre.

Kolb, D. (1984). *Experiential Learning: Experience as the Source of Learning and Development*. Prentice Hall.

Kyriacou, C. (1993). Research on the development of expertise in classroom teaching during initial teacher training and the first year of teaching. *Educational Review*, **45**, 78–88.

L'Aiguille, Y. (1994). Pushing back the boundaries of personal experience. In *Reflective Practice in Nursing* (A. Palmer, S. Burns and C. Bulman, eds) pp. 85–99. Blackwell Scientific Publications.

Landgrebe, B. and Winter, R. (1994). 'Reflective' writing on practice: professional support for the dying? *Educational Action Research*, **2**, 83–94.

Langford, G. (1978). *Teaching as a Profession: an Essay in the Philosophy of Education*. Macmillan.

Langford, M. (1995). Competence and clinical aspiration: the situation for complementary therapies outside the 'big five'. *Complementary Therapies in Medicine*, **3**, 16–20.

Law, H. (1984). *The Uses and Abuses of Profiling*. Harper and Row.

Lomax, P. (1995). Action research for professional practice. *British Journal of In Service Education*, **21**, 49–57.

Lucas, P. (1991). Reflection, new practices, and the need for flexibility in supervising student teachers. *Journal of Further and Higher Education*, **15**, 84–93.

Macmillan (1995). Reflective Practice: the Impact on Patient Outcomes. A conference held at the Commonwealth Institute, 2 November 1995 (comments from the floor).

McIntyre, D. (1989). Criterion-referenced assessment of teaching. In *Rethinking Appraisal and Assessment* (H. Simons and J. Elliot, eds) pp. 64–71. Open University Press.

McIntyre, D. (1994). Classrooms as learning environments for beginning teachers. In *Collaboration and Transition in Initial Teacher Training* (M. Wilkin and D. Sankey, eds) pp. 81–93. Kogan Page.

McIntyre, D. and Haggar, H. (1993). Teachers' expertise and models of mentoring. In *Mentoring: Perspectives on School-based Teacher Education* (D. McIntyre, H. Haggar and M. Wilkin, eds) pp. 86–102. Kogan Page.

McKay, E. and Ryan, S. (1995). Clinical reasoning through story telling: examining a student's case story on a fieldwork placement. *British Journal of Occupational Therapy*, **58**, 234–238.

McLaughlin, T. H. (1994). Mentoring and the demands of reflection. In *Collaboration and Transition in Initial Teacher Training* (M. Wilkin and D. Sankey, eds) pp. 151–160. Kogan Page.

McPherson, H. (1993). The path to mastery: a role for supervision. *European Journal of Oriental Medicine*, **1**, 6–11.

McPherson, H. (1995). Great talents ripen late. *European Journal of Oriental Medicine*, **1**, 35–39.

Mangan, P. (1995). NVQ solution. *Nursing Times*, **91**, 66–68.

Mansfield, B. (1989). Competence and standards. In *Competency-based Education and Training* (J. Burke, ed.) pp. 26–38. Falmer Press.

Mattingly, C. and Fleming, M. (1994). *Clinical Reasoning: Forms of Inquiry in Therapeutic Practice*. F. A. Davis Co.

Maynard, T. and Furlong, J. (1993). Learning to teach and models of mentoring. In *Mentoring: Perspectives on School-based Teacher Education* (D. McIntyre, H. Haggar and M. Wilkin, eds) pp. 69–85. Kogan Page.

Mickan, S. (1995). Student preparation for paediatric fieldwork. *British Journal of Occupational Therapy*, **58**, 239–244.

Mitchell, L. (1989). The definition of standards and their assessment. In *Competency-based Education and Training* (J. Burke, ed.) pp. 54–64. Falmer Press.

National Health Service Executive (1994). *Testing the Vision: a Report on Progress in the First Year of 'A Vision for the Future'*. DoH.

National Health Service Executive (1995). *Clinical Supervision – a Resource Pack*. DoH.

National Health Service Management Executive (1993a). *The A to Z of Quality*. DoH.

National Health Service Management Executive (1993b). *A Vision for the Future*. DoH.

Nias, J. (1987). *Seeing Anew: Teachers' Theories of Action*. Deakin University.

Nisbitt, R. E. and Ross, L. (1980). *Human Inference in Strategies and Shortcomings of Social Judgement*. Prentice Hall.

Osterman, K. and Kottcamp, R. (1993). *Reflective Practice for Educators: Improving Schooling through Professional Development*. Corwin Press Inc.

Palmer, A., Burns, S. and Bulman, C. (1994). *Reflective Practice in Nursing*. Blackwell Scientific Publications.

Passmore, J. (1980). *The Philosophy of Teaching*. Duckworth Press.

Pickering, M. (1987). Interpersonal communication in the supervisory process. In *Supervision in Communication Disorders* (M. Crago and M. Pickering, eds). College Hill Publications.

Pinar, W. (1986). 'Whole, bright and deep with understanding': issues in qualitative research and autobiographical method. In *Recent Developments in Curriculum Studies* (P. Taylor, ed.) pp. 3–18. National Foundation for Educational Research (NFER)/Nelson.

Pollard, A. and Tann, S. (1987). *Reflective Teaching in the Primary School*. Cassell.

Rankin-Box, D. (1995). Competence in clinical settings: issues in nursing practice. *Complementary Therapies*, **3**, 25–27.

Reason, P. (1995). Complementary practice at Phoenix Surgery: first steps in cooperative inquiry. *Complementary Therapies*, **3**, 37–41.

Reed, J. and Procter, S. (eds) (1995). *Practitioner Research in Health Care: the Inside Story*. Chapman and Hall.

Robb, A. and Murray, R. (1992). Medical humanities in nursing: thought provoking? *Journal of Advanced Nursing*, **17**, 1182–1187.

Royal College of Nursing (1995). *The Systematic Development of Guidelines for Good Practice: Standards for Nutritional Care of the Older Adult*. RCN.

Rudduck, J. (1992). Practitioner research and programmes of initial teacher education. In *Teachers and Teaching: from Classrooms to Reflection* (T. Russell and H. Munby, eds) pp. 156–170. Falmer Press.

Rudduck, J. and Hopkins, D. (eds) (1985). *Research as a Basis for Teaching: Readings from the Work of Lawrence Stenhouse*. Heinemann.

Russell, T. (1989). Documenting reflection-in-action in the classroom: searching for appropriate methods. *Qualitative Studies in Education*, **2**, 277–284.

Russell, T. (1993a). Teachers' professional knowledge and the future of teacher education. *International Analysis of Teacher Education, Journal of Teacher Education*, **19**, 205–215.

Russell, T. (1993b). Critical attributes of a reflective teacher: Is agreement possible? In *Conceptualising Reflection in Teacher Development* (J. Calderhead and P. Gates, eds) pp. 144–153. Falmer Press.

Russell, T. and Munby, H. (1991). Reframing: the role of experience in developing teachers' professional knowledge. In *The Reflective Turn: Case Studies in and on Educational Practice* (D. A. Schön, ed.) pp. 164–187. College Teachers Press.

Russell, T. and Munby, H. (eds) (1993). *Teachers and Teaching: from Classroom to Reflection*. Falmer Press.

Ryan, S. (1995). Teaching clinical reasoning to occupational therapists during fieldwork education. In *Clinical Reasoning in the Health Professions* (J. Higgs and L. Jones, eds). Butterworth-Heinemann.

Schön, D. A. (1983). *The Reflective Practitioner*. Basic Books.

Schön, D. (1987). *Educating the Reflective Practitioner*. Jossey Bass.

Schuller, T. (ed.) (1995). *The Changing University?* Open University Press.
Schwab, J. (1969). The practical: a language for the curriculum. *School Review*, November, 1–23.
Scott, P. (1995). *The Meaning of Mass Higher Education*. Open University Press.
Shaw, R. (1992). *Teacher Training in the Secondary School*. Kogan Page.
Shifrin, K. (1993). Setting standards for acupuncture training – a model for complementary medicine. *Complementary Therapies in Medicine*, 1, 91–95.
Shifrin, K. (1995). Squaring the circle: the core syllabus of the British Acupuncture Accreditation Board. *Complementary Therapies in Medicine*, 3, 13–15.
Shulman, L. S. (1987). Knowledge and teaching: foundations of the new reform. *Harvard Educational Review*, 57, 1–22.
Simons, H. and Elliott, J. (eds) (1989). *Rethinking Appraisal and Assessment*. Open University Press.
Smith, J. P. (1995). Clinical supervision: conference organized by NHSME on 29.11.94 at Solihull, England. *Journal of Advanced Nursing*, 21, 1029–1031.
Smith, R. (1992). Theory: an entitlement to understanding. *Cambridge Journal of Education*, 22, 387–398.
Smith, R. and Alred, G. (1993). The impersonation of wisdom. In *Mentoring: Perspectives on School-based Teacher Education* (D. McIntyre, H. Haggar and M. Wilkin, eds) pp. 103–116. Kogan Page.
Sparrow, S. and Robinson, J. (1994). Action research: an appropriate design for research in nursing? *Educational Action Research*, 2, 347–356.
Squirrell, G., Gilroy, P., Jones. D. and Rudduck, J. (1990). *Acquiring Knowledge in Initial Teacher Education*. Library and Information Research Report No. 79, The British Library.
Stengelhofen, J. (1993). *Teaching Students in Clinical Settings*. Chapman and Hall.
Stenhouse, L. (1975). *An Introduction to Curriculum Research and Development*. Heinemann.
Steward, B. (1994). Researching fieldwork practice in occupational therapy. *Educational Action Research*, 2, 259–265.
Stones, E. (1992). *Quality Teaching: a Sample of Cases*. Routledge.
Stronach, I. (1989). A critique of the 'new assessment': from currency to carnival? In *Rethinking Appraisal and Assessment* (H. Simons and J. Elliott, eds) pp.161–179. Open University Press.
Strong, J., Gilbert, J., Cassidy, S. *et al.* (1995). Expert clinicians' and students' views on clinical reasoning in occupational therapy. *British Journal of Occupational Therapy*, 58, 119–122.
Swain, G. (1995). *Clinical Supervision: the Principles and Process*. HVA.
Thow, M. and Murray, R. (1991). Medical humanities in physiotherapy: education and practice. *Physiotherapy*, 77, 733–736.
Titchen, A. and Binnie, A. (1993). A unified action research strategy in nursing. *Educational Action Research*, 1, 25–33.
Tripp, D. (1993). *Critical Incidents in Teaching: Developing Professional Judgement*. Routledge.
Twinn, S. (1989). Change and Conflict in Health Visiting Practice: dilemmas in

the assessment of the competence of student health visitors. (PhD Thesis) London University Institute of Education, unpublished.

Twinn, S. (1992). Issues in the supervision of health visiting practice: an agenda for debate. In *Clinical Supervision and Mentorship in Nursing* (T. Butterworth and J. Faugier, eds) pp. 132–159. Chapman and Hall.

Twinn, S. and Davis, S. (1996). The supervision of Project 2000 students in the clinical setting: issues and implications for practitioners. *Journal of Clinical Nursing*, 5, 177–183.

United Kingdom Central Council for Nursing, Midwifery and Health Visiting (1986). *Project 2000: A New Preparation for Practice*. UKCC.

United Kingdom Central Council for Nursing, Midwifery and Health Visiting (1992a). *The Scope of Professional Practice*. UKCC.

United Kingdom Central Council for Nursing, Midwifery and Health Visiting (1992b). *Code of Professional Conduct*. UKCC.

United Kingdom Central Council for Nursing, Midwifery and Health Visiting (1995a). *The Council's Proposed Standards for Incorporation into Contracts For Hospital and Community Health Care Services*. UKCC.

United Kingdom Central Council for Nursing, Midwifery and Health Visiting (1995b). *Prep and You*. UKCC.

United Kingdom Central Council for Nursing, Midwifery and Health Visiting (1996a). *Position Statement on Clinical Supervision for Nursing and Health Visiting*. UKCC.

United Kingdom Central Council for Nursing, Midwifery and Health Visiting (1996b). *Guidelines for Professional Practice*. UKCC.

Van Manen, M. (1990). Beyond assumptions: shifting the limits of action research. *Theory into Practice*, 30, 152–157.

Van Manen, M. (1995). On the epistemology of reflective practice. *Teachers and Teaching: Theory and Practice*, 1, 9–23.

Walker, R. (1985). *Doing Classroom Research: a Handbook for Teachers*. Methuen.

Walker, R. (1986). The conduct of educational case studies: ethics, theory and procedures. In *Controversies in Classroom Research* (M. Hammersley, ed.) pp. 187–219. Open University Press.

Walsh, M. and Ford, P. (1989). *Nursing Rituals: Research and Rational Actions*. Butterworth-Heinemann.

Watkins, C. (1992). An experiment in mentor training. In *Mentoring in Schools* (M. Wilkin, ed.) pp. 97–115. Kogan Page.

Webb, C. (1993). Action research: philosophy, methods and personal experiences. In *Nursing Art and Science* (A. Kitson, ed.) pp. 120–133. Chapman and Hall.

White, E., Riley, E., Davies, S. and Twinn, S. (1994). *A Detailed Study of the Relationships between Teaching, Support, Supervision and Role Modelling in Clinical Areas, within the Context of the Project 2000 Courses*. ENB.

White, R. and Ewan, C. (1991). *Clinical Teaching in Nursing*. Chapman and Hall.

Wilkin, M. and Sankey, D. (eds) (1994). *Collaboration and Transition in Initial Teacher Training*. Kogan Page.

Wilkin, P. (1992). Clinical supervision in community psychiatric nursing. In

Clinical Supervision and Mentorship in Nursing (T. Butterworth and J. Faugier, eds) pp. 185–199. Chapman and Hall.

Williams, R. (1965). *The Long Revolution*. Pelican.

Wilson, J. (1993). *Reflection and Practice: Teacher Education and the Teaching Profession*. The Althouse Press, University of Western Ontario.

Winter, R. (1989). Teacher appraisal and the development of professional knowledge. In *Quality Teaching: Arguments for a Reflective Profession* (W. Carr, ed.) pp. 183–199. Falmer Press.

Wood, P. (1987). Life histories and teacher knowledge. In *Educating Teachers: Changing the Nature of Pedagogical Knowledge* (J. Smyth, ed.) pp. 121–135. Falmer Press.

Wragg, E. C. (1993). *Classroom Observation*. Cassell.

Zeichner, K. and Liston, D. (1987). Teaching student teachers to reflect. *Harvard Educational Review*, **57**, 23–48.

Index

196   *Index*